Biological Effects of Low Dose Radiation

Biological Effects of Low Dose Radiation

Proceedings of the International Meeting on Biological Effects of Low Dose Radiation held in Cork, Ireland, on 25–26 July 1999

Editors:

Takeshi Yamada
Central Research Institute of Electric
Power Industry CRIEPI
Tokyo, Japan

Carmel Mothersill
Radiation Science Centre
Dublin Institute of Technology
Dublin, Ireland

Barry D. Michael
Gray Laboratory Cancer Research Trust
Mount Vernon Hospital
Northwood, Middlesex, U.K.

Christopher S. Potten
Epithelial Biology Department
Paterson Institute for Cancer Resaerch
Christie Hospital NHS Trust
Manchester, U.K.

2000

ELSEVIER

Amsterdam – London – New York – Oxford – Paris – Shannon – Tokyo

ELSEVIER SCIENCE B.V.
Sara Burgerhartstraat 25
P.O. Box 211, 1000 AE Amsterdam, The Netherlands

First edition 2000

Library of Congress Cataloging in Publication Data
A catalog record from the Library of Congress has been applied for.

ISBN: 0444 50431 1
ISSN: 0531 5131
International Congress Series No. 1211

♾ The paper used in this publication meets the requirements of ANSI/NISO Z39.48-1992 (Permanence of Paper).

Printed in the Netherlands

Preface

This book is derived from a satellite meeting of the 11th International Congress of Radiation Research 1999, entitled "Biological Effects of Low-Dose Radiation" and held in Cork, Ireland on July 25–26, 1999. The meeting was sponsored jointly by the Radiation Science Centre of the Dublin Institute of Technology and the Central Research Institute of the Electric Power Industry, Tokyo, Japan. This book also includes papers by authors from many different parts of the world, which is welcome because the problems of the biological effects of low-dose radiation are universal and require the dedicated attention of leading scientists everywhere.

Risk assessment is fundamental to the protection of public health from radiation exposure, but any estimate of risk is subject to numerous major uncertainties. In view of the uncertainties surrounding the shape of dose-response curves at low levels of ionizing radiation, the linear nonthreshold dose-response model is now widely accepted as a paradigm in radiation protection practice and risk analysis. However, interest among scientists in obtaining a more conclusive understanding of the effects of low-level radiation has been evident in recent initiatives, including a reassessment by the US National Academy of Science of the latest research evidence on the risks of low-level radiation, begun in 1998. Also, a 10-year US Department of Energy research program, begun in the fiscal year of 1999, has been specifically addressing the effects of low-level radiation within human cells, in part to help verify or disprove the linear model. A vigorous worldwide effort is now apparently underway to understand the basic mechanisms underlying the biological effects of low-dose radiation. This book presents a series of papers representing the progress going on, which will undoubtably make an important contribution to this field of research.

I wish to thank the participants in the meeting for their substantial contributions and their participation in the spirited discussion which followed. I would also like to thank Drs Carmel Mothersill, Hiroshi Tanooka, Christian Streffer, Barry D. Michael and Roland Masse for their essential input as members of the Organising Committee of the meeting. Finally, I wish to thank the staff of Elsevier Science Publishers for their efficient cooperation in the production of these proceedings.

Takeshi Yamada

Contents

Cancer and epidemiology

Microdosimetry

The dual response to low-dose irradiation: induction vs. prevention of DNA damage

L.E. Feinendegen[1], V.P. Bond[2] and C.A. Sondhaus[3]

[1] *Nuclear Medical Department, Clinical Center, National Institutes of Health, Bethesda, Maryland;*
[2] *Research Faculty, Washington State University, Richland, Washington; and* [3] *Department of Radiology and Radiation Control Office, University of Arizona, Tucson, Arizona, USA*

Abstract. Ionizing radiation causes damage to DNA that is apparently proportional to absorbed dose (D), yet is still a weak carcinogen. Spontaneous DNA damage in unirradiated cells arises mainly from endogenous reactive oxygen species (ROS), and from environmental toxins. It is presumably the main cause of spontaneous carcinogenesis, despite the qualitative differences in the damage produced. Cells and tissues protect against DNA damage physiologically at various levels of intervention: by damage prevention, repair and removal, e.g., by ROS detoxification, DNA repair, and removal of cells with DNA damage. Ionizing radiation also induces ROS, and mainly alters intracellular signaling at cell doses below about 0.3 Gy, and to a decreasing extent above this dose. This may induce physiological protection against DNA damage lasting from hours to weeks. In analyzing published low-dose effects three questions appear to be pertinent: 1) What is a low dose in terms of cell exposure? 2) What are the cellular responses at low doses? 3) What does this mean in the generation of biological tissue effects? This analysis considers both the damaging and protective radiation effects at low doses. The resulting net dose-risk function strongly suggests that the incidence of cancer is less likely to be proportional to dose than to exhibit a threshold, or even to fall below the spontaneous incidence, when cell doses are below about 0.2 Gy.

Keywords: dual response to low-dose irradiation.

Introduction

Following exposure to ionizing radiation, damage to the DNA of the affected cells may cause cell death and late effects such as malignant tumors. These effects have been studied mainly after absorbed doses above about 0.3 Gy. In humans acutely irradiated above this dose, the risk of cancer in these exposed individuals appears to be proportional to dose [1].

In living cells and tissues low-dose induced DNA changes are less readily observed. Acute and temporary metabolic changes predominate and have been measured at even less than 0.01 Gy [1–4]. These include stimulation of radical detoxification and DNA repair, removal of damaged cells through apoptosis, and activation of an immune response. These activating stimuli do not necessarily appear at high doses. They tend to protect cells and tissues against the production and accumulation of DNA changes, whether they are caused endog-

Address for correspondence: Dr Ludwig E. Feinendegen, Wannental 45, 88131 Lindau/B, Germany.
Tel.: +49-8382-75673. Fax: +1-301-496-0114. E-mail: feinendegen@gmx.net

enously or by radiation [5].

The designation of a "low" dose is physically and operationally vague, although some effect-based guidelines have been suggested. In attempting to analyze both the occurrence and the consequences of low-dose effects in exposed tissues, the doses to individual cells and equivalent micromasses of tissue are fundamentally important. Three questions arise in this regard:

1. What is a "low" dose in terms of cellular exposure?
2. What are the cellular responses to low cell doses?
3. How do these cellular responses relate to the biological effects of low-dose irradiation in tissues and organs?

Cellular exposure at low doses in tissue

Ionizing radiation may affect cells both by direct energy deposition events and through so-called "bystander effects" induced by irradiated neighboring cells (and possibly, to a lesser degree, by irradiated matrix). The probability of both direct and indirect routes depends on the distribution and size of the radiation-induced energy deposition events (also called "hits") in the tissue micromasses. To aid in evaluating the effects of differing absorbed doses in tissues, the hetero-geneity of the energy deposition events, and their sizes at these tissue doses, need to be considered.

The passage of penetrating ionizing radiation through matter results in the deposition of energy from particle tracks that arise stochastically throughout [6]. At sufficiently large absorbed doses, the cells and equivalent micromasses of the exposed tissue are traversed by very large numbers of charged particles; thus, the total energy deposited in a single cell or equivalent micromass, here denoted by "cell-dose", is unlikely to differ much from the tissue absorbed dose (D). As D decreases, the number of energy depositing events in each cell is reduced. When it falls far enough below a mean value of 1 per micromass, the individual cell or micromass will only receive a cell dose that is either 0, or the amount deposited in a single event. The latter is denoted by the term microdose, formally specific energy z_1 [6], with its mean being $\bar{z}_1$. Hence, one, or a multiple of micro-doses, constitutes a cell dose. The mean number of hits per exposed micromasses in which microdoses occur is then $D/\bar{z}_1$. Absorbed dose, D, is thus the ratio of the number of hits of all sizes, N_H, to the number of exposed micromasses, N_e, multiplied by the mean microdose $\bar{z}_1$:

$$D = \bar{z}_1(N_H/N_e) \tag{1}$$

Several aspects derive from Eqn. (1) and should be emphasized as follows:

1. The absorbed dose, D, is the average concentration of energy absorbed per unit mass of tissue, but at sufficiently low values of D, energy is deposited only in some of the micromasses in the exposed tissue. Thus, at low levels, the absorbed dose to the tissue does not describe the varying doses to its cells

or equivalent micromasses, and should not be related to single cell effects.

2. In the lowest dose region, the cell doses are a constant frequency distribution of single microdoses specific to a given radiation quality; that is, $\bar{z}_1$ remains constant for a given radiation. The only variable which increases with dose is then the fraction of micromasses affected, N_H/N_e.

3. High linear energy transfer (LET) radiation produces larger microdoses (higher $\bar{z}_1$), so that fewer hits (lower N_H) will deliver the same D as low LET radiation [7]. Thus, $\bar{z}_1$ and N_H/N_e are inversely related to each other, and the ratios between $\bar{z}_1$ and different values of D are specific to different radiation qualities.

It has been proposed [6] that a low dose be defined as one unlikely to produce more than a single hit in any individual micromass. This condition is roughly met when the fraction of exposed micromasses that are hit is less than or equal to 0.2. From Eqn. (1), this will be true when the absorbed dose, D, is less than one-fifth of the average microdose $\bar{z}_1$. Since a cell may be viewed as a living whole with its structural and functional components interacting through signaling networks, the sensitive target is taken to be the cell, with a spherical volume of average micromass 1 ng [8]. (The averaging of the mass over all cell types follows the practice used in calculations for radiation protection.) Using this value, a dose, D, of 250 kVp X-rays with $\bar{z}_1 = 0.09$ cGy would need to be below about 0.02 cGy to be called "low". In contrast, an absorbed dose as high as 7 cGy would be "low" for 4 MeV alpha particles, where $\bar{z}_1 = 35$ cGy. Using this single hit criterion, that which is considered a low tissue dose is seen to depend on the microdose values, and thus, to vary with radiation quality. In other words, a low tissue dose is much higher at high LET than at low LET. For most purposes, absorbed doses below about 20 cGy may be considered as low.

It can be shown that the dose rate in tissue consists of repeated hits to its micromasses. According to Eqn. (1), during exposure to a radiation field the dose rate, D, per unit time, t, is:

$$D/t = \bar{z}_1(N_H/N_e)(1/t)$$

or:

$$D/t = \bar{z}_1/(t\, N_e/N_H) \tag{2}$$

From Eqn. (1), the denominator (t N_e/N_H) is equal to (t$\bar{z}_1$/D). It gives the average time interval between two consecutive hits per exposed micromass [7,8]. This time interval allows the affected cell to respond acutely, and may be long enough for a second hit not to interfere. Only single or protracted exposures are considered here, in which (t N_e/N_H) is sufficiently long for acute cellular responses and repair to occur without interference from a second hit. For instance, a low-LET background radiation of 1 mGy per year causes about 1 hit per micromass per year.

Cellular responses to low cell doses

It can be postulated that the risk of cancer (R), i.e., the cancer incidence for a given irradiated tissue type, is proportional to the ratio of the number of radiation-induced cancers, N_q, to the number of exposed micromasses, N_e.

The conventionally used macroscopic dose-risk function for organs and tissues following low-dose or dose rate exposure is:

$$R = \alpha D \tag{3}$$

where α is a constant for a given radiation and tissue. Substituting R for the ratio N_q/N_e and D using Eqn. (1), and subsequently multiplying each side by N_e, results in the following equation:

$$N_q = \alpha \bar{z}_1 N_H \tag{4}$$

This equation expresses the incidence of detriment, not as a function of energy absorbed per mass, but as a function of absorbed energy in terms of the number of microdoses. The conventionally used dose-risk function in Eqn. (3) has been transformed into a "hit-number-effectiveness function" at the cellular level [9]. This change to cellular focus provides a new approach to studying low-dose effects. The term N_q can denote, for example, a malignant cell transformation causing a lethal tumor, which is a result of various cellular responses affecting the corresponding DNA change.

"Spontaneous" carcinogenesis causes about 25% of the population in industrialized countries to die from cancer. It is assumed to be due to DNA changes that are mainly endogenous, i.e., metabolically induced by the action of reactive oxygen species (ROS) or by environmental toxins. It may also result, to a minute degree, from thermal instability of DNA, causing spontaneous errors in DNA replication [10—13]. In contrast, radiation-induced carcinogenesis is relatively rare. The corresponding DNA changes may differ qualitatively from endogenous changes, and occur by both direct and indirect actions of ionizing radiation [14—16]. The incidence of such changes appears to be a linear function of dose.

Both spontaneous and radiation-induced carcinogenesis need to be considered in the analysis of cell responses to low doses. The reason for this is, on the one hand, the relatively large extent of spontaneously occurring DNA damage [11—13,17—19], and, on the other hand, the potential additive, as well as protective, effect of low-dose irradiation on this background damage.

Radiation-induced generation of DNA damage

Radiation-induced primary DNA alterations appear to increase linearly with dose, and deviations from linearity in living cells and tissues are usually attributed to secondary biological interventions. Cell doses above about 0.3 Gy, which can occur from single hits (microdoses) to individual cells at low doses of high-LET radiation, may also cause DNA alterations [20,21], as well as gene activation [22] in nonhit cells by so-called clastogenic factors (probably involving ROS) [23]. It is not known whether these bystander effects also occur from cell doses well below 0.3 Gy. Carcinogenesis also appears to be linked with radiation-induced genetic instability [24,25], which increases chromosomal abnormalities and somatic mutations in the descendent cell population over many generations. The overall probability of a carcinogenic cell transformation leading to a lethal tumor has been estimated to be about 10^{-14} per 1-mGy hit per oncogenic human stem cell. This estimate has been based on data from the atomic bomb survivors in Japan assuming linear correspondence between radiation-induced leukemia incidence and absorbed dose; an estimated 10^9 blood-forming stem cells per person; and a mean energy deposition event per ng of 1 mGy [5].

Radiation-induced protection against DNA damage

In different cells and tissues, cell doses of less than 0.2 Gy of low-LET radiation have been readily observed to (relatively slowly) induce acute and reversible metabolic reactions linked to temporary stimulation of cellular protection against various toxic agents, including radiation [1—4]. These adaptive responses involve: 1) detoxification of ROS, 2) induction of DNA repair, and 3) removal of damaged cells by both apoptosis and stimulated immune response, as indicated in Fig. 1.

Detoxification of ROS
Low tissue doses of low-LET radiation, even below 0.01 Gy, have been found to alter intracellular metabolism in mouse bone marrow for a period of about 10 h [2]. The change was shown to involve a temporary depression of the enzyme thymidine kinase to a minimum at about 4 h postirradiation and a concomitant elevation of nonbound glutathione indicating an increased ROS detoxification [26—30]. Similar results in different tissues of rodents have been reported from

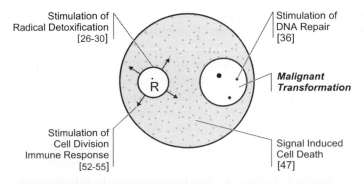

Stimulation of Radical Detoxification [26-30]

Stimulation of DNA Repair [36]

R

Malignant Transformation

Stimulation of Cell Division Immune Response [52-55]

Signal Induced Cell Death [47]

Fig. 1. Summary of low-dose specific cellular responses (single or few hits).

various laboratories. Low doses temporarily reduced the uptake of the thymidine analogue 5-iodo-2-deoxyuridine (IUdR) into cellular DNA for up to 24 h [31]. Low doses increased the activity of glutathione [32] and of superoxide dismutase (SOD), with a concomitant reduction in the rate of membrane oxidation in exposed brain tissues for a period of weeks [33]. The low-dose induced elevation of glutathione resulted in protection against drug-induced lipid peroxidation in mouse liver [34].

Induction of DNA repair

Low-dose induced protection of human lymphocytes against chromosomal aberrations from subsequent high-dose irradiation has indicated a stimulation of DNA repair. This protective effect reached its maximum at about 4 h and extended to about 60 h after the conditioning low-dose irradiation [35—38]. Moreover, low doses protected against somatic mutations [39] and against spontaneous oncogenic transformation in cell culture [40,41]. Low-dose induced DNA repair was demonstrated in tissue culture cells, with an ultrasensitive assay for in vivo DNA damage that occurs both endogenously and after irradiation [42]. Genetic instability in culture cells was also seen to be reduced by low-dose irradiation [43]. The various mechanisms of protection may be directly or indirectly linked with the transient activation of different genes, including those involved in ROS detoxification and in controlling cell cycle check points [44—46].

Removal of damaged cells

Low doses of low-LET radiation may induce removal of damaged cells from tissue through apoptosis. Depending on cell type, its incidence was found to rise in a linear or curvilinear relation to dose, even including the possibility of a low-dose induced reduction [47—49]. Above about 0.1 Gy, apoptosis incidence appeared to rise with a slope of around $5 \cdot 10^{-3}$ per mGy [49]. In mouse spleen cells, induction of apoptosis appeared to be maximal at 4 h after 0.5 Gy X-irradiation, with a return to normal values within about 24 h [50]. In different culture cell lines, all of which were radioresistant at high doses, increased lethality at doses of at most 0.2—0.4 Gy was implicated as being associated with an induction of radioresistance at higher doses [51]. Apoptosis obviously expresses elimination of radiation-induced DNA damage by what has been called "altruistic cell suicide" [47].

A second principal mode of removal appears to operate through low-dose induced stimulation of cellular immune competence. The latter has been observed to peak at about 0.1—0.2 Gy, beyond which the stimulation rapidly disappeared and immune failure increased. These responses were shown to last for several weeks in whole-body irradiated rodents [1,52—55]. In another study, the incidence of lung and lymph node metastases significantly decreased 1 week after 0.2 Gy whole body γ-irradiation of tumor-bearing rats. At the same time, the proportion of $CD8^+$ cells and lymphocytes that infiltrate the tumor tissue significantly increased; and the transcription of the genes for IFN-γ and tumor necrosis factor α (TNF-α) in spleen and tumor tissue had also increased, whereas that for Tgfb was decreased [56].

Low-dose induced cellular protection disappearing at high doses

In the case of ROS detoxification, a quantitative relation between dose and degree of protection has been developed using, in a first step, single whole-body gamma irradiation of mice resulting in average cell doses from <0.01 to 1 Gy [5,57]. The activity of thymidine kinase and uptake of the thymidine analogue IUdR in bone marrow cells consistently reached a dose-dependent minimum at 4 h (as discussed above). When the low-dose irradiated mice were again irradiated at 4 h with tissue doses of 0.01 or 0.1 Gy, the depressed thymidine kinase activity and IUdR uptake both rapidly reverted to a normal level [28]. The degree of this reversion by renewed irradiation declined when the second dose was larger than about 0.1 Gy; and reversion did not occur above 0.5 Gy [5,56].

The above dose-response relation agrees in principle with studies on lymphocytes. For example, the incidence of chromosomal aberrations in low-dose irradiated human lymphocytes in vitro first declined with increasing dose to below the background level; the aberration incidence only increased with doses above 0.05 Gy [58]. In particular, it has been found that single low-LET radiation doses below, but not above, about 0.2 Gy may condition human lymphocytes in vitro to become protected against chromosomal aberrations after high-dose irradiation [35—37,59—61]. This phenomenon appears to be linked to stimulated DNA repair.

With regard to the removal of damaged cells, apoptosis in mouse thymocytes was significantly reduced below background level at 24 h after single low-LET irradiation with up to about 0.2 Gy, and the incidence of apoptosis only rose with higher doses in a linear fashion [48]. Immune competent cells providing immune protection in rodents were stimulated over several weeks, following single doses up to about 0.1- to 0.2-Gy low-LET radiation; immune inhibition only occurred after doses higher than about 0.2 Gy [52—55].

Gene activation is probably involved in the inverse dose-response function that has been reported for various radioresistant cell lines. They have shown an increased mortality rate at single low-LET low doses, with a maximum at about 0.2 to 0.4 Gy, after which resistance to radiation took over [51]. The expression of the c-jun gene in tissue culture cells also responded to low doses, D, of low- but not high-LET radiation; the latter, of course, results in high cell doses compared with low-LET radiation [62]. In line with this, the thioredoxin gene reached its maximal expression in liver cells after 0.25—0.5 Gy, with a decline to levels below control after higher doses of low-LET radiation [45]. This gene is involved in the de novo synthesis of glutathione and also plays a more general role in activating various genes including the c-jun gene. On the other hand, the transient activation of the glutathione reductase gene in liver cells increased with dose, at least up to 1 Gy [45].

Despite the limited number of observations, which are summarized in Table 1,

Table 1. Low-dose response disappearing at high doses.

Response	Reference	D (Gy) maximum response
Radical detoxification		
Prot. TdR-K (BM cells)	[10]	0.1
Ind. SOD (mitoch. brain)	[33]	0.5
DNA damage reduction		
Red. Chr. Ab. (lymph.)	[58]	0.05
Prot. Chr. Ab. (lymph.)	[59]	0.2
DNA damage removal		
Ind. immune comp.	[52]	0.1
	[54]	0.1
	[55]	0.1
Apoptosis (thymocytes)	[48]	0.15
Apoptosis (culture cells)	[51]	0.2—0.4
Gene expression		
c-fos (culture cells) ↑	[64]	0.25
c-jun, -myc, -Ha-ras (culture cells) ↑	[64]	0.5
DIR1 (human epith. cells) ↓	[65]	0.2
Thioredoxin (liver cells) ↑	[45]	0.2—0.5

low cell doses with a maximum around 0.1—0.2 Gy appear to cause a particular set of protective responses lasting from hours to weeks, depending on species, individual organism, cell type, and components of the DNA damage-control mechanisms. These responses are confined to low cell doses, disappear at higher doses, and are easily measured. This dose-response curve contrasts with the linear dose-effect curve for radiation-induced DNA damage, as shown in Fig. 2. The relatively low incidence of radiation-induced DNA damage at low doses suggests that the protective responses primarily affect the production and/or accu-

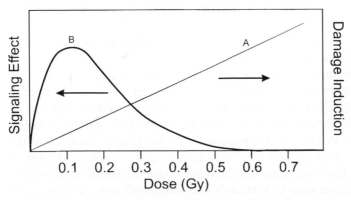

Fig. 2. The two dose response curves for radiation-induced generation of DNA damage **(A)** and prevention of DNA damage **(B)**.

mulation of more abundant endogenous DNA damage. The DNA repair processes usually observed after high doses are apparently more robust than those protective mechanisms that are initiated in cells by low doses [10,63].

Cellular responses to low doses in causing tissue effects

The tissue effects described above appear as a composite of cellular responses [64]. Because $\bar{z}_1$ in Eqn. (4) is a constant for a given radiation quality, the proportionality constant α expresses the biological effect in the irradiated system over a certain range of N_H. On the cell level, however, α appears to include the competing probabilities of damaging and protective responses in the exposed tissue. A plausible way in which these probabilities appear to combine on the cell and tissue level, based on the experimental results reviewed in the previous section, is accordingly outlined in the following summary. It indicates their relative influence on the kind of low-level dose-response relation that an increasing body of evidence appears to support.

In this discussion, the probability per average hit of a given radiation that induces a malignant tumor in a specific tissue is assigned the term p_{ind}. It is considered to be constant at approximately 10^{-14} per average hit from low-LET radiation in human hemopoietic stem cells, as discussed above [5].

The value of p_{ind} may be enhanced, for example, by way of genetic instability [24,25]. The degree of enhancement is denoted here by p_{enh}. It is not known whether p_{enh} is appreciable at cell doses below about 0.2 Gy, but it is likely larger than p_{ind}. The product $p_{ind} \cdot p_{enh}$ may be a constant at low doses. Because of the extremely low p_{ind}, the product $p_{ind} \cdot p_{enh}$ will still remain comparatively small. The value of p_{enh} is taken here to be negligible at low doses.

The probability of spontaneous oncogenic transformation in a human hemopoietic stem cell leading to a lethal leukemia is denoted here by p_{spo}; it is estimated to be approximately 10^{-11} over an individual's life span [5].

The probability of cellular protection appears to vary with dose; it appears to be relatively high at low doses and to disappear with high doses, as discussed above. The low-dose specific protective responses may be estimated quantitatively by their overall effect on reducing fixed DNA damage (that is caused mainly by endogenous sources). This cumulative probability then expresses the degree of protection against fixed DNA damage per cell per average hit, p_{prot} [5,57]. Thus, an $N_H \cdot p_{prot}$ value of 0.2 means a 20% reduction of fixed cellular DNA damage. To indicate its dose dependence (as discussed above) p_{prot} is here denoted by $p_{prot}(D)$. In contrast to p_{ind} and p_{spo}, $p_{prot}(D)$ is transient. Hence, the assignment of different p values needs to allow for the differences in the time during which they act. One way to do so is to adjust $p_{prot}(D)$ by a factor dividing the average duration of $p_{prot}(D)$ by the average time span from cellular oncogenic transformation step to tumor development, assuming proportionality between fixed DNA damage and cancer development [5]. For example, suppose an $N_H \cdot p_{prot}(D)$ of 0.2 lasts an average of 10 days, and the average time span between cellular oncogenic transformation and tumor development is 5 years, i.e., 1,825 days. Then, the time-corrected value of $N_H \cdot p_{prot}(D)$, now denoted by $N_H \cdot p_{prot}(D,t)$, is 0.2 (10/1825) = $\sim 10^{-3}$.

Other corrections may be required to account for as yet unknown confounding factors. For instance, protection may also be triggered as well as suppressed by intercellular communication including bystander effects; otherwise it would not be observed so easily at low doses. A few of the confounding factors may perhaps eventually be evaluated for a given cell system; but, whatever the mechanisms involved may be, the results of protection, i.e., less DNA damage or a lower probability of cancer, are measurable. Thus, the term $p_{prot}(D,t)$ expresses the cumulative probability of protection against DNA damage and the resulting cancer induction from both irradiation and endogenous causes (p_{ind} and p_{spo}). The value of p_{spo} will be orders of magnitude larger than that of p_{ind}.

Regardless of the mechanisms involved, the p values will undoubtedly vary with the species, individual organism, cell type, and microdose. Therefore, as in the model below, p_{ind}, p_{enh}, and $p_{prot}(D,t)$ need to be determined for the same radiation quality, corresponding to the average microdose and cell type (from the same individual). This includes the possibility that the various responses are triggered indirectly by hits in cell-free matrix and through bystander effects [20,21].

Thus, with:

p_{spo} = lifetime probability of spontaneous oncogenic transformation and cancer development, per cell

p_{ind} = probability of radiation-induced oncogenic transformation and cancer development, per average hit

p_{enh} = fractional enhancement of p_{ind}, per average hit

$p_{prot}(D,t)$ = cumulative probability of protection against fixed DNA damage and cancer in tissue, i.e., against p_{spo}, p_{ind}, and p_{enh}, per average hit

the number of cancers, N_q, induced by low doses in the exposed tissue can now be related to N_H as follows:

$$N_q = [p_{ind} + p_{ind} \cdot p_{enh} - p_{prot}(D,t) \cdot p_{spo} - p_{prot}(D,t) \cdot p_{ind} - p_{prot}(D,t) \cdot p_{ind} \cdot p_{enh}] N_H \tag{5}$$

Combining Eqns. (4) and (5):

$$\alpha = [p_{ind} (1 + p_{enh}) - p_{prot}(D,t) (p_{spo} + p_{ind} + p_{ind} \cdot p_{enh})]/\bar{z}_1 \tag{6}$$

and solving for R in Eqn. (3):

$$R = [p_{ind} (1 + p_{enh}) - p_{prot}(D,t)(p_{spo} + p_{ind} + p_{ind} \cdot p_{enh})] D/\bar{z}_1 \tag{7}$$

The value of p_{ind} is comparatively smaller than p_{spo}, and p_{enh} is considered to be zero at low doses of low-LET radiation. Therefore, substituting ($D/\bar{z}_1$) for the term (N_H/N_e) from Eqn. (1); Eqn. (7) may be simplified to:

$$R = [p_{ind} - p_{prot}(D,t) \cdot p_{spo}] \, (N_H/N_e) \tag{8}$$

From the above, the value of α does not appear to be constant at low doses over the range of D in which the value of $p_{prot}(D,t)$ decreases against p_{ind} with increasing D, i.e., N_H. However, at higher doses of low-LET radiation, and, consequently, with higher cell doses the term $p_{prot}(D,t)$ disappears and α becomes constant.

Concerning the term α for high-LET radiation, the corresponding relatively high values of $\bar{z}_1$ may make $p_{prot}(D,t)$ ineffective in the hit cells. However, p_{ind}, $p_{ind} \cdot p_{enh}$, and p_{spo} may be offset by $p_{prot}(D,t)$, if protective mechanisms are initiated in nonhit cells by intercellular signal substances and specific clastogenic factors stemming from irradiated cells. Such intercellular stimuli must be considered to affect nonhit cells in both ways, i.e., both inducing damage and signaling for protective responses. Besides induction of chromosomal aberrations, induction of genes, such as that coding for the p53 protein, has been observed as a bystander effect [22]. ROS may be involved in this phenomenon [23].

Figure 3 summarizes the model based on Eqn. (8). The dashed line shows $(N_H/N_e)(p_{ind})$, the increase in cancer above background levels due to radiation if there were no protective mechanisms. The background line shows the spontaneous cancer incidence p_{spo}, most of which is due to endogenous DNA alterations, mainly from normal cellular metabolism. The light solid line indicates the radiation-induced reduction in spontaneous cancer incidence, $(N_H/N_e)[p_{prot}(D,t) \cdot p_{spo}]$. The heavy solid line shows the combined effects of cancer induction and prevention, i.e., the net dose-risk function, R, in Eqn. (8). The shaded region represents

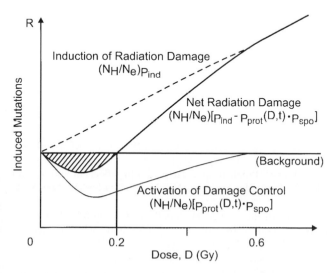

Fig. 3. Schematic diagram combining the potential dual effects and indicating a probable deviation from linearity with a hormetic effect at low doses (see text for details). Mutations: mis/unrepaired DNA alterations.

the possible reduction of cancer incidence due to protective effects; this has been termed "radiation hormesis". The "threshold" shown for observable radiation-induced cancer, 0.2 Gy, agrees with various epidemiological data [1,3,4].

Only statistically significant changes in R after exposure of mammalian populations to low-LET radiation below 0.2 Gy may determine whether detrimental or beneficial effects predominate. Indeed, several sets of epidemiological and experimental data tend to support the existence of a threshold, or even of beneficial (hormetic) effects at low doses and low-dose rates of low-LET radiation [1,3,4]. It needs to be seen to what degree adaptive responses are initiated in multicellular systems exposed to very low doses of high-LET radiation, or to individually high cell doses.

Acknowledgements

The authors express their deep appreciation to the late Dr K.I. Altman, Department of Biochemistry and Biophysics, University of Rochester Medical Center, Rochester, New York, for a long and fruitful collaboration; to Dr E.P. Cronkite, Brookhaven National Laboratory, Upton, New York, Dr M. Frazier, Office of Biological and Environmental Research of the US Department of Energy, Washington, DC, Dr R.D. Neumann, Department of Nuclear Medicine, Clinical Center, National Institutes of Health, Bethesda, Maryland, and Dr M. Pollycove, US Nuclear Regulatory Commission, Rockville, Maryland, for their encouragement, support, valuable discussions and editorial help; and Mrs B. MacMahon and J. Rochek for careful secretarial assistance.

This research was supported in part by the US Department of Energy under contract No. DE-AC02-76H00016.

References

1. UNSCEAR. Sources and Effects of Ionizing Radiation, Annex B: Adaptive Responses to Radiation in Cells and Organisms. New York: United Nations, 1994.
2. Zamboglou N, Porschen W, Muehlensiepen H, Booz J, Feinendegen LE. Low-dose effect of ionizing radiation on incorporation of iodo-deoxyuridine into bone marrow cells. Int J Radiat Biol 1981;39:83—93.
3. Sugahara T, Sagan LA, Aoyama T (eds). Low-Dose Irradiation and Biological Defense Mechanisms. Amsterdam, London, New York, Tokyo: Excerpta Medica, 1992.
4. Academie des Sciences, Institut de France. Problems associated with the effects of low doses of ionizing radiations. Rapport de l'Academie des Sciences, No. 38. Paris, London, New York: Lavoisier, TecDoc, 1995.
5. Feinendegen LE, Loken M, Booz J, Muehlensiepen H, Sondhaus CA, Bond VP. Cellular mechanisms of protection and repair induced by radiation exposure and their consequences for cell system responses. Stem Cell 1995;13(1):7—20.
6. ICRU (Intational Commission on Radiation Units and Measurements). Microdosimetry, Report 36. Bethesda, Maryland, USA: ICRU, 1983.
7. Feinendegen LE, Booz J, Bond VP, Sondhaus CA. Microdosimetric approach to the analysis of cell responses at low dose and low dose rate. Radiat Prot Dosim 1985;13:299—306.

8. Feinendegen LE, Bond VP, Booz J. The quantification of physical events within tissue at low levels of exposure to ionizing radiation. ICRU News 1994;2:9—13.

9. Bond VP, Benary V, Sondhaus CA, Feinendegen LE. The meaning of linear dose-response relations, made evident by use of absorbed dose to the cell. Health Phys 1995;68:786—792.

10. Friedberg EC, Walker GC, Siede W. DNA Repair and Mutagenesis. Washington DC, USA: ASM Press, 1995.

11. Ames BN, Gold LS, Willet WC. The causes and prevention of cancer. Proc Natl Acad Sci USA 1995;92:5258—5265.

12. Beckman KD, Ames BN. Oxidative decay of DNA. J Biol Chem 1997;272:19633—19636.

13. Helbock HJ, Beckman KB, Shigenaga MK, Walter PB, Woodall AA, Yeo HC, Ames BN. DNA oxidation matters: the HPLC-electrochemical detection assay of 8-oxo-deoxyguanosine and 8-oxo-guanine. Proc Natl Acad Sci USA 1998;96:288—293.

14. Ward JF, Blakely WJ, Joner EI. Mammalian cells are not killed by DNA single-strand breaks caused by hydroxyl radicals from hydrogen peroxide. Radiat Res 1985;103:383—392.

15. Ward JF. DNA produced by ionizing radiation in mammalian cells: identities, mechanisms of formation, and reparability. Prog Nucl Acid Res Mol Biol 1988;35:95—125.

16. Wallace SS. Enzymatic processing of radiation-induced free radical in DNA. Radiat Res 1998; 150(5, Suppl):60—79.

17. Feinendegen LE, Bond VP, Sondhaus CA, Altman KI. Cellular signal adaptation with damage control at low doses vs. the predominance of DNA damage at high doses. Comput Rend Acad Sci Paris Life Sci 1999;322:245—251.

18. Pollycove M, Feinendegen LE. Molecular biology, epidemiology, and the demise of the linear no-threshold (LNT) hypothesis. Comput Rend Acad Sci Paris Life Sci 1999;322:197—204.

19. Feinendegen LE. The role of adaptive responses following exposure to ionizing radiation. Hum Exp Toxicol 1999;18:426—432.

20. Nagasawa H, Little JB. Induction of sister chromatid exchanges by extremely low doses of alpha particles. Cancer Res 1992;52:6394—6396.

21. Emerit I, Oganesian N, Sarkisian T, Arutyunyan R, Pogosian A, Asrian K, Levy A, Cernjavski L. Clastogenic factors in the plasma of Chernobyl accident recovery workers: anticlastogenic effect of Ginkgo biloba extract. Radiat Res 1995;144:198—205.

22. Azzam EL, de Toledo SM, Gooding T, Little JB. Intercellular communication is involved in the bystander regulation of gene expression in human cells exposed to very low fluence of alpha particles. Radiat Res 1998;150:497—504.

23. Narayanan PK, Goodwin EH, Lehnert BE. Alpha particles initiate biological production of superoxide anions and hydrogen peroxide in human cells. Cancer Res 1997;57:3963—3971.

24. Morgan WF, Day JP, Kaplan MI, McGhee EM, Limoli CL. Genomic instability induced by ionizing radiation. Radiat Res 1996;146:247—258.

25. Meydan D, Hellgren D, Lambert B. Variations in the frequency of the T cell receptor beta/gamma-interlocus recombination in long-term cultures of nonirradiated and X- and gamma-irradiated human lymphocytes. Int J Radiat Biol 1998;74:697—703.

26. Feinendegen LE, Muehlensiepen H, Lindberg C, Marx J, Porschen W, Booz J. Acute and temporary inhibition of thymidine kinase in mouse bone marrow cells after low-dose exposure. Int J Radiat Biol 1984;45:205—215.

27. Feinendegen LE, Muehlensiepen H, Bond VP, Sondhaus CA. Intracellular stimulation of biochemical control mechanisms by low-dose low-LET irradiation. Health Phys 1987;52:663—669.

28. Feinendegen LE, Bond VP, Booz J, Muehlensiepen H. Biochemical and cellular mechanisms of low-dose effects. Int J Radiat Biol 1988;53:23—37.

29. Laval F. Pretreatment with oxygen species increases the resistance of mammalian cells to hydrogen peroxide and gamma rays. Mutat Res 1988;201:73—79.

30. Hohn-El-Karim K, Muehlensiepen H, Altman KI, Feinendegen LE. Modification of effects of radiation on thymidine kinase. Int J Radiat Biol 1990;58:97—110.

31. Misonoh J, Yoshida M, Okumura Y, Kodama S, Ishii K. Effects of low-dose irradiation of X-rays

on IUDR incorporation into mouse tissues. In: Sugahara T, Sagan LA, Aoyama T (eds) Low-Dose Irradiation and Biological Defense Mechanisms. Amsterdam, London, New York, Tokyo: Excerpta Medica, 1992;323—326.

32. Kojima S, Matsuki O, Kinoshita I, Gonzalet Valdes T, Shimura N, Kubodera A. Does small-dose gamma ray radiation induce endogenous antioxidant potential in vivo? Biol Pharmacol Bull 1997;20:601—604.

33. Yamaoka K, Edamatsu R, Mori A. Effects of low-dose X-ray irradiation on old rats — SOD activity, lipid peroxide level, and membrane fluidity. In: Sugahara T, Sagan LA, Aoyama T (eds) Low-Dose Irradiation and Biological Defense Mechanisms. Amsterdam, London, New York, Tokyo: Excerpta Medica, 1992;419—422.

34. Kojima S, Matsuki O, Kubodera A, Yamaoka K. Elevation of mouse liver glutathione level by low-dose gamma ray irradiation and its effect on CCl_4-induced liver. Anticancer Res 1998;18: 2471—2476.

35. Olivieri G, Bodycote J, Wolff S. Adaptive response of human lymphocytes to low concentrations of radioactive thymidine. Science 1984;223:594—597.

36. Wolff S, Afzal V, Wienke JK, Olivieri G, Michaeli A. Human lymphocytes exposed to low doses of ionizing radiations become refractory to high doses of radiation as well as to chemical mutagens that induce double-strand breaks in DNA. Int J Radiat Biol 1988;53(1):39-49.

37. Wolff S. The adaptive response in radiobiology: evolving insights and implications. Environ Health Perspect 1998;106(1):277—283.

38. Ikushima T, Aritomi H, Morisita J. Radioadaptive response: efficient repair of radiation-induced DNA in adapted cells. Mutat Res 1996;358:193—198.

39. Rigaud O, Papadopoulo D, Moustacchi E. Decreased deletion mutation in radioadapted human lymphoblasts. Radiat Res 1993;133:94—101.

40. Azzam EI, de Toledo SM, Raaphorst GP, Mitchel REJ. Low-dose ionizing radiation decreases the frequency of neoplastic transformation to a level below the spontaneous rate in C3H 10T1/2 cells. Radiat Res 1996;146:369—373.

41. Redpath JL, Antoniono RJ. Introduction of an adaptive response against spontaneous neoplastic transformation in vitro by low-dose gamma radiation. Radiat Res 1998;149:517—520.

42. Le XC, Xing JZ, Lee J, Leadon SA, Weinfeld M. Inducible repair of thymine glycol detected by an ultrasensitive assay for DNA. Science 1998;280:1066—1069.

43. Suzuki K, Kodama S, Watanabe M. Suppressive effect of low-dose preirradiation on genetic instability induced by X-rays in normal human embryonic cells. Radiat Res 1998;150:656—662.

44. Boothman DA, Meyers M, Odegaard E, Wang M. Altered G_1 checkpoint control determines adaptive survival responses to ionizing radiation. Mutat Res 1996;358:143—153.

45. Kojima S, Matsuki O, Nomura T, Kubodera A, Honda Y, Honda S, Tanooka H, Wakasugi H, Yamaoka K. Induction of mRNAs for glutathione synthesis-related proteins in the mouse liver by low doses of gamma rays. Biochim Biophys Acta 1998;1381:312—318.

46. Tubiana M. Effets cancerogenes des faibles doses du rayonnement ionisant. Radioprotection 1996;31:155—191.

47. Kondo S. Health Effects of Low-Level Radiation. Osaka, Japan: Kinki University Press; and Madison, Wisconsin, USA: Medical Physics Publishing, 1993.

48. Shu-Zheng L, Yin-Chun Z, Ying M, Xu S, Jian-Xiang L. Thymocyte apoptosis in response to low-dose radiation. Mutat Res 1996;358:185—191.

49. Ohyama H, Yamada T. Radiation-induced apoptosis: a review. In: Yamada T, Hashimoto Y (eds) Apoptosis, its Roles and Mechanisms. Tokyo, Japan: Business Center for Academic Societies Japan, 1998;141—186.

50. Fujita K, Ohtomi M, Ohyama H, Yamada T. Biphasic induction of apoptosis in the spleen after fractionated exposure of mice to very low doses of ionizing radiation. In: Yamada T, Hashimoto Y (eds) Apoptosis, its Roles and Mechanisms. Tokyo, Japan: Business Center for Academic Societies Japan, 1998;201—218.

51. Joiner MC, Lambin P, Malaise EP, Robson T, Arrand JE, Skov KA, Marples B. Hypersensitivity

to very low single radiation doses: its relationship to the adaptive response and induced radio-resistance. Mutat Res 1996;358:171—183.

52. James SJ, Makinodan T. T cell potentiation by low-dose ionizing radiation: possible mechanisms. Health Phys 1990;59:29—34.

53. Makinodan T. Cellular and subcellular alteration in immune cells induced by chronic, intermittent exposure in vivo to very low dose of ionizing radiation (ldr) and its ameliorating effects on progression of autoimmune disease and mammary tumor growth. In: Sugahara T, Sagan LA, Aoyama T (eds) Low-Dose Irradiation and Biological Defense Mechanisms. Amsterdam, London, New York, Tokyo: Excerpta Medica, 1992;233—237.

54. Anderson RE. Effects of low-dose radiation on the immune response. In: Calabrese EJ (ed) Biological Effects of Low-Level Exposures to Chemicals and Radiation. Chelsea, Michigan: Lewis Publishers Inc., 1992;95—112.

55. Sakamoto K, Myojin M, Hosoi Y, Ogawa Y, Nemoto K, Takai Y, Kakuto Y, Yamada S, Watabe N. Fundamental and clinical studies on cancer control with total or upper half body irradiation. J Jpn Soc Ther Radiol Oncol 1997;9:161—175.

56. Hashimoto S, Shirato H, Hosokawa M, Nishioka T, Karamitsu Y, Matushita K, Kobayashi M, Miyasaka K. The suppression of metastases and the change in host immune response after low-dose total-body irradiation in tumor-bearing rats. Radiat Res 1999;151:717—1724.

57. Feinendegen LE, Bond VP, Sondhaus CA, Muehlensiepen H. Radiation effects induced by low doses in complex tissue and their relation to cellular adaptive responses. Mutat Res 1996;358:199—205.

58. Pohl-Rueling J, Fischer P, Haas O. Effect of low-dose acute X-irradiation on the frequencies of chromosomal aberrations in human peripheral lymphocytes in vitro. Mutation Res 1983;110:71—82.

59. Shadley JD, Wolff S. Very low doses of X-rays can induce human lymphocytes to become less susceptible to ionizing radiation. Mutagenesis 1987;2:95—96.

60. Shadley JD, Wienke JK. Induction of the adaptive response by X-rays is dependent on radiation intensity. Int J Radiat Biol 1989;56:107—118.

61. Shadley JD, Dai G. Cytogenetic and survival adaptive responses in G_1 phase human lymphocytes. Mutat Res 1992;265:273—281.

62. Woloschak GE, Chang-Liu C-M. Effects of low-dose radiation on gene expression in Syrian hamster embryo cells: comparisons of Janus neutrons and gamma rays. In: Sugahara T, Sagan LA, Aoyama T (eds) Low-Dose Irradiation and Biological Defense Mechanisms. Amsterdam, London, New York, Tokyo: Excerpta Medica, 1992;239—242.

63. Kleczkowska H, Althaus FR. The role of poly(ADP-ribosyl)ation in the adaptive response. Mutat Res 1996;358:215—221.

64. Feinendegen LE. Radiation risk of tissue late effect, a net consequence of probabilities of various cellular responses. Eur J Nucl Med 1991;18:740—751.

65. Prassad AV, Mohan N, Chandrasekar B, Meltz ML. Induction of transcription of "immediate early genes" by low-dose ionizing radiation. Radiar Res 1995;143:263—272.

66. Robson T, Price ME, Moore ML, Joiner MC, McKelveu-Martin VJ, McKeown SR, Hirst DG. Increased repair and cell survival in cells treated with DIR1 antisense oligonucleotides: implications for induced radioresistance. Int J Radiat Biol 2000;76:617—623.

Energy barriers for radiation-induced cellular effects

Antone L. Brooks, Edmond E. Hui and Victor P. Bond

Environmental Sciences, Washington State University Tri-Cities, Richland, Washington, USA

Abstract. The linear-no-threshold (LNTH) hypothesis states that a single radiation-induced ionization may result in an increased risk of cancer. Implied is that any amount of energy deposited in a system increases the risk. All-or-nothing changes can be defined as quanta responses, which can be added. These should be related to extensive physical quantities, which can also be summed. In this report, the net number of induced quantal biological changes is plotted against total energy imparted to the system. Dose (Gy), an intensive quantity that is dependent on mass, is replaced with energy (Joules), an extensive quantity that is independent of mass. With this approach, it is possible to define energy barriers below which no significant increase in the frequency of mutations, chromosome aberrations, or cancer can be demonstrated. If the LNTH is valid at low doses, the efficiency for the production of quantal changes must remain constant. It is demonstrated that the energy required to induce quantal changes increases as the dose decreases. The presence of energy barriers and the change in efficiency for production of quantal changes suggest that the LNTH does not hold at very low doses. These observations may be useful in the standard setting for occupational exposures.

Keywords: cancer, chromosome aberrations, energy barriers, linear-no-threshold hypothesis, mutations.

Introduction

The linear-no-threshold hypothesis (LNTH) suggests that single ionization can produce an increased level of biological damage. This hypothesis does not take into account several important biological factors. First, there is a background level for biological changes such as mutations, chromosome aberrations and cancer. To induce an increase in these quantal responses above that background level, it is necessary to produce a level of damage that can be detected. Second, the LNTH assumes that the amount of biological damage is linearly dependent on total radiation dose and that the efficiency for producing damage is constant at all levels of radiation dose. If there are cell/cell or cell/matrix interactions that change as a function of the fraction of the cell population that is damaged, the efficiency for production of the damage may change as a function of dose. This paper is designed to evaluate these factors and conduct a test of two hypotheses that could impact the LNTH. These hypotheses are:

Address for correspondence: Antone L. Brooks, Washington State University Tri-Cities, 2710 University Drive, Richland, WA 99352, USA. Tel.: +1-509-372-1912. Fax: +1-509-372-1204.
E-mail: tbrooks@tricity.wsu.edu

1. There are energy barriers below which no significant increase in the frequency of quantal responses above the background level can be identified.
2. The amount of energy required per excess quantal response remains constant as a function of radiation dose.

Methods

Data sets from well-defined biological systems were evaluated to test these hypotheses. The background level of damage was subtracted from the total response, so that the responses being evaluated were the net number of quantal responses observed. Next, the system was defined as the number of cells or units evaluated for each of the dose groups. The dose was then multiplied by the number of cells or units involved in detection of the quantal responses. This results in a number that reflects the amount of energy required to produce the response if the mass of the cells or units is known. It was not possible to know the exact mass and distribution of masses in the biological populations evaluated. Thus, mass was not included in these calculations and so the values used are not a direct measure of the energy deposited in the defined system, but are directly proportional to energy.

To test the first hypothesis, the net number of radiation-induced responses was related to the energy deposited in the system. From this it was possible to make an estimate of the energy barrier below which responses were not observed. This approach made it possible to determine if such an energy barrier exists for the endpoint of primary concern, the induction of cancer in humans.

To test the second hypothesis on the efficiency of the energy for induction of quantal responses, the amount of energy was divided by the net number of quantal responses induced and plotted as a function of the radiation dose. This approach provides a test of the efficiency of producing quantal responses. It also defines the amount of energy needed in the system to induce each of the quantal responses measured. If the doses are restrained to the low-dose region, so that most of the cells are in the single-hit response range of the dose-response relationship, and if a constant amount of energy would be needed to produce each quantal response regardless of total radiation dose, then the LNTH would be supported.

In these studies, the data sets evaluated represent different levels of biological organization. We first analyzed the data on the induction of mutations in *Tradescantia* [1]. This data set was selected because of the wide range of radiation doses used and the wide range of different cell numbers evaluated to detect changes in the total mutations induced. Next, data sets which demonstrated changes in the frequency of radiation-induced chromosome aberrations were studied [2,3]. These were selected based on the large cell population sizes and dose ranges evaluated. The Pohl-Ruling et al. data [2] represent an attempt to detect the induction of chromosome aberrations after exposure to very small doses. In these studies the number of cells scored was held rather constant (about 9,000 cells per dose group) and a wide range of different doses used to detect changes in aberration frequency. This study illustrates the consequences of decreasing the amount of energy in the system by holding the size of the cell population constant. Studies were conducted where the researchers increased the number of cells scored as the dose decreased, but did not attempt to detect increased levels of chromosome aberrations at very low radiation doses [3]. Thus, they worked in a region where they had an increase in aberration frequency at all doses since they tried to maintain a rather constant amount of energy in the system as they decreased the dose. From these data it was possible to evaluate the efficiency of the energy deposited in the production of the aberrations and test the second hypothesis. Finally, the data from the atomic bomb survivors were used to determine if the observations made at the cellular and molecular level may be applicable to human data for radiation induced cancer [4,5].

From the evaluation of these data sets it was possible to test our two hypotheses.

Results

The data for the *Tradescantia* are plotted in Fig. 1 and provide an estimation of the relative amount of energy in each of the defined dose groups required to induce excess mutations. In this graph, the dose (cGy) to each group is listed next to each data point. This figure illustrates that as the dose was decreased from 48 to 6 cGy, the amount of energy put into the system decreased, since the number of stamen hairs scored at each dose group was relatively constant. Scoring about 3,000 stamen hairs exposed to a dose of 6 cGy demonstrated that it

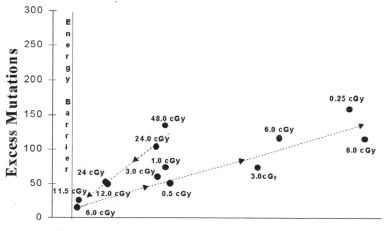

Energy (Stamen hairs x Dose x Mass/hair)

Fig. 1. Demonstration of an energy barrier for induction of mutations in *Tradescantia*. Excess mutations are plotted as a function of energy. From [1].

was not possible to detect a significant excess number of induced mutations. There were 17 mutations in 3,374 stamen hairs scored in the exposed cells as compared to 11 mutations in 3,525 stamen hairs scored in the control cells. Additional dose groups were then defined with larger cell populations and exposed to the same or to lower total radiation doses (6.0, 3.0, 1.0, 0.5 and 0.25 cGy). The experiment was designed to increase the number of stamen hairs scored for each of the dose groups to a level calculated to result in a significant increase in net number of mutations. For the low-dose groups, when the amount of energy deposited in these defined cell populations was related to the net number of mutations induced, large amounts of energy had to be added to the system to induce the additional mutations. The slope of the line that describes the energy-mutation relationships at lower doses has a lower slope than observed following exposure to higher radiation doses. This graph illustrates that there is a definite energy barrier below which it is not possible to detect an increase in the net number of mutations. For this experimental system, it seems that the barrier is located where $\sim 3,000$ cells were exposed to 6 cGy. This energy barrier can only be invaded by either decreasing the dose or decreasing the number of stamen hairs scored or by varying both the dose and the number of stamen hairs scored. Any of these will result in a product that is equal to or less than that observed when 3,000 cells were scored after exposure to 6 cGy. This product of dose and cell numbers result in an estimate of the total energy in the system. Anything that lowers the energy to the system will lower the level of response (net mutations). Thus, the barrier cannot be invaded. In attempts to go to lower doses and test the LNTH, the scientists evaluating mutations in *Tradescantia* increased the number of stamen hairs evaluated to increase the net number of mutations. However, with the increased number of stamen hairs scored, the total energy to the new system was increased, again leaving the energy barrier intact.

A publication on the induction of chromosome aberrations illustrates an example of a data set where the dose continued to be decreased below the energy barrier and the number of cells remained rather constant [2]. The total energy is plotted against the net number of chromosome aberrations in Fig. 2. This plot shows that the level of aberrations does not increase above the background level for all the dose levels below about 10 cGy. When the number of excess mutations is plotted against excess aberrations there is an apparent plateau for the data below 5 cGy. To get an excess number of chromosome aberrations, it would have been necessary to increase the number of cells scored by at least a factor of two for the cGy point. However, in doing this, the amount of energy in the system would have been the same as the cells exposed to 10 cGy. This is another way of demonstrating that there is indeed an energy barrier below which it is not possible to observe an increase in the number of quantal responses.

Studies were conducted to determine if the same logic could be applied to the survivors of the atomic bomb [4,5]. In these data sets, the number of individuals were varied as a function of the dose and exposure, so that at the low-dose groups there were larger numbers of individuals represented. For radiation-induced leu-

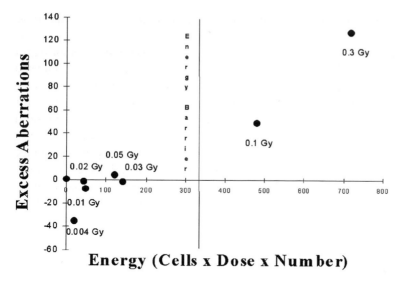

Fig. 2. Demonstration of an energy barrier for the induction of chromosome aberrations in human blood lymphocytes. Excess chromosome aberrations are plotted as a function of energy. From [2].

kemia, there is not a significant increase in the number of cancers observed until the dose level increased above 0.2–0.5 Sv [4]. Therefore, the energy barrier is rather high (Fig. 3).

For the total solid tumors the number of excess tumors was related to the total amount of energy in the total population. The amount of energy required to produce tumors at the two lowest doses was higher than that required at the higher

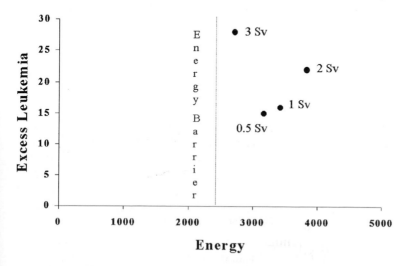

Fig. 3. Demonstration of an energy barrier for the induction of leukemia in A-bomb survivors. Excess leukemia is plotted as a function of energy. From [4].

doses. Thus, although the energy barrier is not well-established it seems to be present [5].

After establishing that there are energy barriers below which no significant increase in quantal responses can be detected, it was important to evaluate the cause of these barriers. One of the potential causes of the barriers is that the efficiency for production of quantal responses decreases as the dose decreases. This was again tested in the well-defined *Tradescantia* data [1]. In Fig. 4, the amount of energy/mutation is plotted against the radiation dose delivered. The energy/mutation should be constant as a function of dose if the LNTH is to hold, since this is a measure of efficiency for mutation production. The Figure illustrates that the amount of energy required to produce a mutation increases as the dose decreases. This suggests that at low doses more energy is required to produce a mutation, thus disproving the second hypothesis. The statement that any amount of energy increases the risk (LNTH) may need to be revised to reflect the fact that as dose decreases the amount of energy required to produce a mutation increases.

To determine if similar patterns of energy per quantal response would hold for other endpoints, we evaluated the amount of energy required to induce chromosome aberrations as a function of radiation dose in Fig. 5 [3]. Again the pattern is the same. At high doses, a rather constant amount of energy is required per chromosome aberration induced. As the dose is decreased, the amount of energy per aberration increases. This pattern again disproves the second hypothesis put forth in this paper and does not support the LNTH. The amount of energy required for each aberration should be constant as a function of radiation dose if the LNTH is to hold.

Finally, it was of interest to evaluate the efficiency for the induction of cancers as a function of total energy deposited in a system. This was done using the

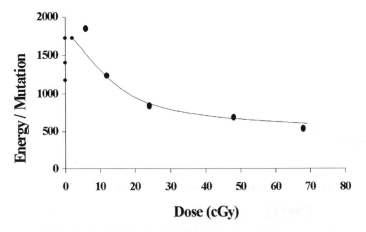

Fig. 4. The efficiency of producing mutations in *Tradescantia*. The amount of energy per excess mutation is plotted as a function of radiation dose. From [1].

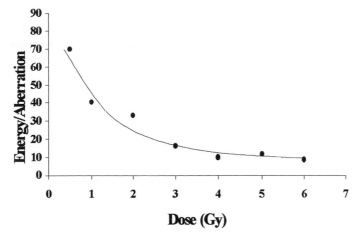

Fig. 5. The efficiency of producing chromosome aberrations in human blood lymphocytes. The amount of energy per excess chromosome aberration is plotted as a function of radiation dose. From [3].

data previously published, plotted in Fig. 6 [5]. Again, the pattern is similar with a rather constant amount of energy required per tumor (3 kJ/cancer) over the higher dose ranges and with an apparent increase in energy required per cancer at the lower radiation doses. As noted, the changes at the lowest doses are not significant [5] and it is difficult to make a very strong argument for this observation. The pattern is similar to that observed for the cellular and molecular end-

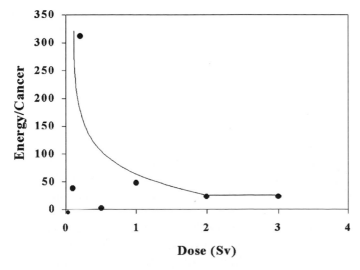

Fig. 6. The efficiency of producing solid tumors in the A-bomb survivors. The amount of energy per excess cancer is plotted as a function of radiation dose. From [5].

points. When a similar evaluation was made for the leukemia data, no excess leukemia was observed in the lowest three groups [4]. From this, one could infer that very large amounts of energy may be required to induce leukemia following exposures to low doses.

Discussion

The apparent energy barriers seem to be related to background level for the endpoint being evaluated, and the amount of energy required to induce the quantal change. If a biological endpoint was being evaluated which had a zero background or spontaneous level of damage, then perhaps it would be possible to argue that any amount of energy added to the system would result in an increase in the measured response. However, biological changes from DNA breakage to cancer all have background levels that are produced by other factors in the environment. This makes energy barriers a "fact of life" for these endpoints, since the product of the dose and the number of subjects evaluated represent the amount of energy required to induce a level of damage that is significantly elevated above the background level. At some low level of energy, it is not possible to define or measure a response that is significantly elevated above the background. This energy level represents the energy barrier. It is not possible to invade the space below such an energy barrier.

If the amount of energy required to produce a quantal response was constant as a function of dose, then one could postulate that the dose required to detect a response could be very small, as long as the population evaluated was very large. However, data reported here suggest that at low doses the amount of energy required to produce these quantal responses (mutations, chromosome aberrations, cancer) increases as dose decreases. This makes it very difficult to detect significant changes regardless of the size of the population evaluated. It is tempting to try to understand the mechanistic basis of these biological observations. For example, it may be possible to postulate that bystander effects [6,7] may be responsible for the observed requirement for an increased amount of energy at lower doses. That is to say that the ratio of damage cells to normal cells must exceed a certain level to be induced with the same efficiency as observed for aberrations, mutations and cancers. If the ratio of damaged cells to normal cells is lower than a certain value, then the normal cells may influence the production of the quantal responses either by induction of apoptosis [8] or induction of repair genes [9] that could result in a form of an adaptive response [10]. Without additional data to provide adequate understanding of the mechanisms involved, this is, of course, speculation.

The fact remains that there are energy barriers below which it is not possible to detect significant levels of biological change. This supports the first hypothesis. We have shown that the efficiency for induction of quantal responses in several biological systems decreased as the dose decreased. This disproves our second hypothesis, which required that the amount of energy to produce responses remains constant as a function of radiation dose. The support of the first hypothesis and the disproof of the second hypothesis suggest that the LNTH is not applicable for induction of biological damage by low doses of low-LET ionizing radiation.

References

1. Sparrow AH, Underbrink AG, Rossi HH. Mutations induced in *Tradescantia* by small doses of X-rays and neutrons: analysis of dose-response curves. Science 1972;176:916—918.
2. Pohl-Ruling J, Fischer P, Haas O, Obe G, Natarajan AT, Buckton KE, Bianchi NO, Larramendy M, Kucerova M, Polikova Z, Leonard A, Farby L, Palitti F, Sharma T, Binder W, Mukerjee RN, Mukerjee U. Effect of low-dose X-irradiation on the frequencies of chromosomal aberrations in human peripheral lymphocytes in vivo. Mutat Res 1983;110:71—82.
3. Bauchinger M, Schmid E, Zitzelsberger H, Braselmann H, Nahrstedt U. Radiation-induced chromosome aberrations analyzed by two-color fluorescence in situ hybridization with composite whole chromosome-specific DNA probes and a pancentromeric DNA probe. Int J Radiat Biol 1993;64(2):179—184.
4. Pierce DA, Y. Shimizu Y, Preston DL, Vaeth M, Mabuchi K. Studies of the mortality of atomic bomb survivors. Report 12, part I. Cancer: 1950—1990. Radiat Res 1996;146:1—27.
5. Bond VP, Benary V, Sondhaus, CA. A different perception of the linear, nonthreshold hypothesis for low-dose irradiation. Proc Natl Acad Sci USA 1991;88:8666—8670.
6. Nagasawa H, Little JB. Induction of sister chromatid exchanges by extremely low doses of alpha particles. Cancer Res 1992;52:6394—6396.
7. Lehnert BE, Goodwin EH. Extracellular factor(s) following exposure to alpha particles can cause sister chromatid exchanges in normal human cells. Cancer Res 1997;57:2164—2171.
8. Limonli CL, Hartmann A, Shephard L, Yang C, Boothman DA, Bartholomew J, Morgan WF. Apoptosis, reproductive failure, and oxidative stress in Chinese hamster ovary cells with compromised genomic integrity. Cancer Res 1998;58:3712—3718.
9. Azzam EI, deToledo SM, Gooding T, Little JB. Intercellular communication is involved in the bystander regulation of gene expression in human cells exposed to very low flounces of alpha particles. Radiat Res 1998;15:497—504.
10. Wolff S. The adaptive response in radiobiology: evolving insights and implications. Environ Health Perspect 1998;106:277—283.

Bystander effect and transformation

A bystander effect of α-particles induces genomic instability in haemopoietic cells

Eric G. Wright

University of Dundee, Department of Molecular and Cellular Pathology, Ninewells Hospital and Medical School, Dundee, Scotland, UK

Abstract. Chromosomal instability has been demonstrated in vitro in the clonal descendants of primary murine and human haemopoietic stem cells after low dose α-irradiation. The instability is transmissible in vivo following transplantation of α-irradiated mouse bone marrow, but its induction has a strong dependence on genetic factors. The induced chromosomal instability may be accompanied by an increased frequency of gene mutations and an increased incidence of apoptosis. These effects, collectively termed radiation-induced genomic instability, are induced at frequencies considerably greater than conventional mutation frequencies. The high frequencies suggest that epigenetic changes may be important and a particular feature of the mechanism(s) underlying the persistence of instability in haemopoietic cells is oxidative stress. In these various investigations there was no dose-response relationship, and instability was demonstrated in the progeny of more cells able to survive being hit by an α-particle than was expected. The expression of instability in the progeny of nonirradiated stem cells has now been formally demonstrated to be due to interactions between irradiated and nonirradiated cells. This type of mechanism (increasingly being recognized in radiobiology) is generally called a bystander effect.

Keywords: genetic predisposition, macrophages, oxidative stress.

Introduction

There is now considerable evidence that the progeny of irradiated cells may express delayed mutational responses including specific gene mutations, a variety of chromosome aberrations, and also exhibit an enhanced death rate (lethal mutations or delayed reproductive death) for many cell divisions postirradiation [1]. These effects are generally regarded as the consequences of a destabilisation of the genome collectively termed radiation-induced genomic instability. Of particular relevance to the issue of low dose effects are those studies that have demonstrated the induction of instability by environmentally relevant doses of α-particles in primary haemopoietic stem cells (the cells from which all blood cells are derived and the target cells for certain radiogenic leukaemias) [2].

A particular feature of α-particle irradiation is that the entire insult is concentrated into a relatively small number of separate, densely ionizing tracks of very limited ranges. At low doses, any individual cell in a tissue is likely to receive no dose,

Address for correspondence: Prof Eric G. Wright, Department of Molecular and Cellular Pathology, University of Dundee, Ninewells Hospital and Medical School, Dundee DD1 9SY, Scotland, UK. Tel.: +44-1383-632169. Fax: +44-1382-633952. E-mail: e.g.wright@dundee.ac.uk

or, if it happens to be in the path of a track, to receive a substantial dose of radiation. The fact that a single traversal of a haemopoietic stem cell will deliver approximately 0.5 Gy to that individual cell [3], and a single traversal of a cell is the lowest possible dose it can receive, emphasises the important distinction between tissue dose and individual cell dose (when discussing low dose α-irradiation).

The first demonstration of α-particle induced genomic instability came from experiments designed to investigate the consequences of irradiating haemopoietic stem cells with low doses of α-particles [4]. In these investigations there was no evidence of a dose-response relationship, and instability was demonstrated in the progeny of more cells (than were theoretically expected) being hit and able to survive (because of the Poisson distribution of α-particles). An explanation of these discrepancies has been provided by more recent experiments [5] in which it was shown that instability can be initiated by a "bystander" mechanism involving interactions between irradiated and nonirradiated cells.

Radiation-induced chromosomal instability and other delayed effects in haemopoietic cells

Using an in vitro clonogenic assay to obtain clonal cell populations derived from haemopoietic stem cells present in α-irradiated cell-suspensions of mouse bone marrow (approximately 1 traversal per cell) it was found that up to half the colonies had nonclonal karyotypic abnormalities, typically involving up to 20% of the metaphases with a high frequency of chromatid-type aberrations [4]. In addition to this chromosomal instability, the cells also exhibited an increased frequency of apoptosis and a 5- to 10-fold increase in nonclonal mutations at the hypoxanthine-guanine-phosphoribosyl-transferase (hprt) locus [6]. Using an assay for comparable human bone marrow clonogenic stem cells, similar chromosomal instability and delayed apoptosis has been demonstrated [7,8]. The results of these studies were interpreted as the high-frequency induction of a lesion in an α-irradiated stem cell resulting in the transmission of chromosomal instability to the progeny of the irradiated cell.

In the studies of human haemopoietic cells chromosomal instability was not induced in all bone marrow samples and it was suggested that this might be attributed to genetic differences between individuals [7]. This interpretation was supported by studies in which bone marrow obtained from different inbred mouse strains [9] could be shown to be susceptible, or relatively resistant to the induction of chromosomal instability. A similar genotype-dependent expression of chromosomal instability has also been demonstrated for γ-irradiated mouse mammary epithelial cells [10]. These studies clearly demonstrate the importance of genetic factors in the predisposition to inducible instability.

To explore the potential in vivo relevance of the chromosomal instability induced in vitro, α-irradiated bone marrow was transplanted into syngeneic mice and a persisting chromosomal instability in haemopoietic cells of donor origin was recorded for up to a year after transplantation [11]. This was interpreted

Table 1. Haemopoietic chromosomal instability persists in vivo in mice transplanted with bone marrow exposed in vitro to 3 Gy X-rays, 0.5 Gy α-particles or 0.5 Gy Californium neutrons.

Months post-transplantation	% Metaphases expressing instability			
	Control	X-rays	α-particles	Neutrons
‹0.5	2	8	4	–	(–)[a]
3–4.5	<1	7	7	5	(4)[a]
6–7.5	<1	2	17	5	(3)[a]
9–12	1	3	6	6	(5)[a]

[a]Data for mice receiving total body neutron irradiation demonstrating the induction in vivo of a persisting instability.

as a long-lived α-particle induced lesion in the repopulated host haemopoietic system (transmitted from the donor repopulating stem cells). This in vivo expression has also been demonstrated in the progeny of stem cells irradiated in vitro with X-rays and neutrons (Table 1). Whilst these transplantation studies facilitate the investigation of the in vivo expression and consequences of the instability phenotype induced by in vitro irradiation, they do not address the question of whether instability can be induced in vivo. More recent studies, however, have demonstrated that by total-body neutron irradiation, a persisting chromosomal instability can be initiated in vivo (Table 1).

Mechanisms underlying α-particle-induced genomic instability

At present little is understood of the mechanism(s) underlying radiation-induced genomic instability, but, in all studies, the various delayed effects of radiation have been demonstrated at frequencies considerably greater than conventional mutation frequencies. These high frequencies, together with the reproducibility of effects, argue against instability being due to mutation of a variety of "genome stability genes". Rather, the data favour the possibility of epigenetic mechanisms.

Under conditions where haemopoietic cells have been shown to exhibit chromosomal instability, the cells demonstrate a wide variety of changes characteristic of oxidative stress [12]. The findings are consistent with oxy-radical metabolism contributing (at least in part) to the persisting chromosomal instability in haemopoietic cells. This suggestion is supported by the observations that bone marrow obtained from the susceptible and resistant mouse strains exhibited different rates of superoxide production following biochemical stimulation [9]. Furthermore, cytogenetic analysis confirmed clastogenic activity in biochemically stimulated cells obtained from a sensitive strain but no significant induction of cytogenetic abnormalities in cells from a resistant strain.

A feature of the induction of chromosomal instability in haemopoietic cells by α-particles is that the proportion of colonies exhibiting instability fails to reflect the expected dose-response relationship (Table 2). Furthermore, if the assump-

Table 2. The significant discrepancy in the observed and expected frequencies of haemopoietic colonies exhibiting chromosomal instability defined by the incidence of nonclonal cytogenetic aberrations. With the grid interposed between the α-particle source and the cells 1 Gy absorbed dose is delivered to the unshielded cells only.

α-irradiation (Gy)	Colonies exhibiting instability	
	Observed	Expected
0.25	2/5 = 0.40	0.06
0.5	22/38 = 0.58	0.11
1.0	45/74 = 0.61	0.20
1.0 with grid	41/63 = 0.65	0.03

tion is made that the maximum expected proportion of stem cells exhibiting instability is equal to the proportion of surviving stem cells traversed by one or more α-particles, then the number of colonies expressing instability is well in excess of the expected value (Table 2). To address the discrepancy in the observed and expected values experimentally, advantage was taken of the Poisson distribution of α-particles to design experiments in which the interposing of a shielding grid between the cells and the source of α-particles resulted in the shielded cells not being irradiated, and the majority of the exposed clonogenic stem cells being killed [5]. Survival data demonstrated that interposing the grid produced the (theoretically) expected reduction in the number of clonogenic cells traversed and killed by α-particles, but there was not the expected 6- to 7-fold reduction in the number of descendant clones exhibiting chromosomal instability (Table 2).

Because experimental conditions of dose, particle fluence, and linear energy transfer were precisely defined in these experiments, it is evident that instability was demonstrated in the progeny of an essentially unirradiated population of clonogenic stem cells. The induction of the instability must be attributed to interactions between irradiated and nonirradiated cells by some mechanism reminiscent of a cytokine-mediated effect. This type of phenomenon is becoming known in radiobiology literature as the "bystander effect".

The demonstration of the induction of instability in the descendants of unirradiated haemopoietic stem cells is at variance with the original interpretation, i.e., of a DNA lesion in a stem cell producing a transmissible chromosomal instability in the progeny of that irradiated cell. Furthermore, the enhanced oxyradical activity in the progeny of irradiated stem cells [12] also points to the potential for indirect mechanisms being important in maintaining, as well as inducing, the phenotype. It is possible that "radiation-activated" accessory cells, most probably phagocytes, have many of the characteristics of the activated macrophages found in inflammatory conditions. Such cells are known to produce clastogenic factors via the intermediacy of superoxide and are able to produce gene mutations, DNA base modifications, DNA strand breaks, cytogenetic damage and transforming events in neighbouring cells [13]. Such activated accessory cells, generated as a consequence of induced instability in vitro or in vivo, may contribute to genetic changes in neighbouring haemopoietic cells (including stem cells). Potentially, such activated phagocytes in vivo may produce genetic damage in nonhaemopoietic cells. The proposal that instability derived activated phagocytes may produce genetic lesions in a variety of neighbouring cells is similar to the mechanisms proposed to explain the relationship between inflammation and carcinogenesis [14], and this has many interesting implications for radiation pathology.

Acknowledgements

The author's research has been supported by the Medical Research Council, The United Kingdom Coordinating Committee on Cancer Research, The Leukaemia Research Fund, The Kay Kendall Leukaemia Fund and the Department of Health. The author acknowledges the members of his laboratory, past and present, who have made important contributions to the emerging story of radiation-induced genomic instability.

References

1. Mothersill C (ed). State of the art report of current research on genomic instability. Int J Radiat Biol 1998;74:663−804.
2. Wright EG. The pathogenesis of leukaemia. In: Hendry JH, Lord BI (eds) Radiation Toxicology: Bone Marrow and Leukaemia. London: Taylor and Francis, 1995;245−274.
3. Lorimore SA, Goodhead DT, Wright EG. Inactivation of haemopoietic stem cell by slow alpha-particles. Int J Radiat Biol 1993;63:655−660.
4. Kadhim MA, Macdonald DA, Goodhead DT, Lorimore SA, Marsden SJ, Wright EG. Transmission of chromosomal instability after plutonium alpha-particle irradiation. Nature 1992;355: 738−740.
5. Lorimore SA, Kadhim MA, Pocock DA, Papworth D, Stevens DL, Goodhead DT, Wright EG. Chromosomal instability in the descendants of unirradiated surviving cells after alpha-particle irradiation. Proc Natl Acad Sci USA 11998;95:5730−5733.
6. Harper K, Lorimore SA, Wright EG. Delayed appearance of radiation-induced mutations at the Hprt locus in murine haemopoietic cells. Exp Hematol 1997;25:263−269.
7. Kadhim MA, Lorimore SA, Hepburn MD, Goodhead DT, Buckle VJ, Wright EG. Alpha-particle induced chromosomal instability in human bone marrow cells. Lancet 1994;344: 987−988.
8. Kadhim MA, Lorimore SA, Townsend KMS, Goodhead DT, Buckle VJ, Wright EG. Radiation-induced genomic instability: delayed cytogenetic aberrations and apoptosis in primary human bone marrow cells. Int J Radiat Biol 1995;67:287−293.
9. Watson GE, Lorimore SA, Clutton SM, Kadhim MA, Wright EG. Genetic factors influencing alpha-particle induced chromosomal instability. Int J Radiat Biol 1997;71:497−503.
10. Ponnaiya B, Cornforth MN, Ullrich RL. Radiation-induced chromosomal instability in BALB/c and C57BL/6 mice. The difference is as clear as black and white. Radiat Res 1997;147: 121−125.
11. Watson GE, Lorimore SA, Wright EG. Long-term in vivo transmission of alpha-particle induced chromosomal instability in murine haemopoietic cells. Int J Radiat Biol 1996;69:175−182.
12. Clutton SM, Townsend KMS, Walker C, Ansell JD, Wright EG. Radiation-induced genomic instability and persisting oxidative stress in bone marrow cultures. Carcinogenesis 1996;17: 1633−1639.

13. Wright EG. Inherited and inducible chromosomal instability: a fragile bridge between genome integrity mechanisms and tumourigenesis. J Pathol 1999;187:19—27.
14. Weitzman SA, Gordon LI. Inflammation and cancer: role of phagocyte-generated oxidants in carcinogenesis. Blood 1990;76:655—663.

©2000 Elsevier Science B.V. All rights reserved.
Biological Effects of Low Dose Radiation.
T. Yamada et al., editors.

Radiation-induced transformation of human cells in vitro

Andrew Riches and Clare Peddie

Medical Science and Human Biology, School of Biology, University of St. Andrews, St. Andrews, Scotland, UK

Abstract. Radiation carcinogenesis has been studied in the past using animal models and in vitro transformation assays. In man, epidemiological surveys have provided useful information, but suitable in vitro models need to be developed to investigate molecular mechanisms. Radiation-induced transformation of human cells in vitro has proved difficult to achieve. Primary cultures cannot be studied for a sufficient length of time and, thus, human cells have to be immortalised to enable studies to be undertaken. Initially, immortalisation was carried out using transection with viral constructs and studies of radiation-induced transformation on human fibroblasts and human epithelial cells are reviewed.

More recently, human epithelial cells were immortalised using a telomerase construct. Using a human retinal pigment the epithelial cell line immortalised in this way, it is now shown that, following exposure to fractionated doses of gamma irradiation, there are marked changes in anchorage-independent growth of these cells. Irradiated cloned cell lines derived from these cultures were tumourigenic in thymic nude mice and exhibited characteristic chromosomal changes.

These human cell lines immortalised with telomerase promise to be useful models in the further investigation of the mechanisms of radiation-induced carcinogenesis.

Keywords: carcinogenesis, epithelial, telomerase.

Initial attempts to investigate and quantify carcinogenic effects of ionizing radiation used in vitro studies of rodent cell lines, in vivo studies using animals, or epidemiological surveys of exposed populations. The C3H10T1/2 clone 8 cell line has been used extensively in radiation-carcinogenesis studies using focus formation as an index of transformation. Similarly the short-term culture of Syrian hamster embryo cells also provided a suitable model to investigate cell transformation, again scoring changed patterns of growth in vitro. In both cases, the assay allows the measurement of cell survival and cell transformation so that transformation frequencies can be determined. It has proved more difficult to develop suitable quantitative models of human carcinogenesis.

Epidemiological studies still provide a valuable means of modelling data on human carcinogenesis. The nature of these studies require careful and time-consuming collection of data.

While rodent cell lines have proved to be useful, they do have a high rate of spontaneous transformation and in most cases are not the key target cell popula-

Address for correspondence: Dr Andrew Riches, Medical Science and Human Biology, School of Biology, Bute Medical Building, University of St. Andrews, St. Andrews KY16 9TS, Scotland, UK. Tel.: +44-1334-463603. Fax: +44-1334-463600. E-mail: A.C.Riches@st-andrews.ac.uk

tion for radiation-induced carcinogenesis. It would obviously be an advantage if studies could be undertaken on human cell populations in vitro.

Human cell systems

As culture methods improved, it became possible to maintain human cells in culture. Organ cultures maintain the three-dimensional relationships of the cell systems, but in general are difficult to establish for extended culture periods. Desegregated cells could be grown in culture but primary strains (in general) underwent senescence after a fixed number of population doubling in vitro. It thus became necessary to immortalise the human cell strains in order for longer-term studies to be utilised. It was then possible to investigate the effects of ionizing radiations on human cells in vitro as summarised in Table 1.

Human fibroblasts

One of the earliest reports of transformation was by Borek [1] who used a human skin fibroblast strain (KD cells). Following irradiation in vitro with a single dose of 4 Gy of X-irradiation, foci formed in vitro. The cells from these foci were shown to exhibit anchorage-independent growth and where tumourigenic in thymic nude mice.

A careful study by Namba et al. [2] demonstrated that transformation could be induced in a human embryo fibroblast strain following repeated exposure to ^{60}Co gamma-irradiation. Little et al. [3] concluded that this was a rare occurrence as they were unable to demonstrate immortalisation in 46 separate experiments, suggesting that immortalisation is the rate-limiting step in transformation of human diploid cells. Cells from a near-diploid human fibroblast cell strain (MSU-1.1) were transformed after a single exposure to ^{60}Co gamma-irradiation [4]. The frequency of transformation was a linear function of radiation dose. Cell lines derived from the foci were tumourigenic in thymic nude mice (8/13). Loss of TP53 activity was not sufficient to cause tumourigenicity as three of the six nontumourigenic foci had also lost all TP53 transactivation function.

A novel approach allowing human cells to be investigated utilised a hybrid cell line between HeLa cells and a human skin fibroblast. This cell line was non-tumourigenic and did not express the cell surface marker: intestinal alkaline phosphatase (IAP). IAP is a radiation-induced tumour-associated antigen and thus forms a useful marker to identify transformed clones [5]. This model allows quantitative measurements of transformation to be made and has recently implicated the loss of alleles on both chromosome 11 and 14 in the radiation-induced neoplastic transformation process [6].

Table 1. Transformation of human cells by ionizing radiations.

Cell type	Origin of cells	Immortalisation procedure	Radiation treatment	Reference
Fibroblast	Primary cell strain human embryo cells	Primary cell strain	^{60}Co gamma	Namba et al. [2]
Fibroblast	Primary cell strain MSU - 1.1	Primary cell strain	^{60}Co gamma	O'Reilly et al. [4]
Fibroblast	Early passage skin fibroblasts	Primary cell strain	X-rays	Borek. [1]
Fibroblast	Skin fibroblast hybrid cell HeLa x fibroblast	Hybrid cell line	Gamma	Redpath et al. [5]
Keratinocyte	Keratinocyte cell line RHEK-1	ad12 - SV40 hybrid virus	X-rays / Fission neutrons	Thraves et al. [7] / Rhim et al. [8] / Thraves et al. [9]
Urothelial cells	Low-grade indolent tumour cell line	SV40	X-rays	Pazzaglia et al. [10]
Bronchial epithelial cells	Bronchial epithelial cell line BEP2D	HPV18	Alpha particles	Hei et al. [11]
Thyroid epithelial cells	Thyroid epithelial cell line HTori-3	SV40 ori$^-$	^{137}Cs gamma / Alpha particles	Riches et al. [14] / Riches et al. [15]
Prostate epithelial cells	Fetal prostate epithelial cell line 267B1	SV40 T antigen	X-rays	Kuettel et al. [13]
Mammary epithelial cells	Primary cell line H185B5	Benzopyrene treated	Heavy ions	Yang et al. [17] / Yang et al. [18]
Mammary epithelial cells	Primary cell culture MEC 76N	Primary cell strain	Gamma	Wazer et al. [19] / Wazer and Band [20]

Human epithelial cells

While studies on fibroblasts are useful, it would be of interest to study human epithelial cells as these are key targets for transformation. Human epithelial cells require immortalisation in order to be studied (in culture) for extended periods of time. Human epidermal keratinocytes were immortalised using an adenovirus type 12 and simian virus 40 construct. Neoplastic progression was thus demonstrated using X-irradiation [7,8] and fission neutrons [9]. The RHEK cell line formed foci in vitro and was tumourigenic in thymic nude mice.

Neoplastic progression was also demonstrated using an SV40 immortalised urothelial cell line. A cell line was produced from a low-grade indolent tumour that was induced following chemical carcinogen treatment. This cell line (SV-HUC MC-T11) progressed to a tumour with more aggressive growth characteristics after exposure to 6 Gy X-irradiation [10]. Chromosome deletions similar to those induced following chemical carcinogen exposure were also observed.

Malignant transformation of human bronchial epithelial cells using radon-simulated α-particles was achieved by using a human bronchial epithelial cell line (BEP2D) that had been immortalised with human papilloma virus (HPV 18) [11,12]. Cells could be transformed with a single dose of 30 cGy of α-particles. The irradiated cells were tumourigenic in thymic nude mice and exhibited anchorage-independent growth. No point mutations at either codon 12/13 or 61 were observed in any of the rash oncogenes (K-, N- and H-rash).

Human prostate epithelial cells immortalised using SV40 T antigen were also studied. Transformation was induced following multiple exposure to 2-Gy X-rays and tumourigenicity was induced in cells that had been further irradiated after selection of anchorage-independent colonies [13]. Accumulated doses of 30 Gy were required to induce tumourigenicity in thymic nude mice. No p53 or rash mutations were detected.

Human thyroid epithelial cells were used as a model of thyroid carcinogenesis in vitro. Cells were immortalised using an SV40 origin minus construct and were transformed following exposure to single or fractionated doses of gamma-irradiation [14] and single doses of alpha-irradiation [15]. The relative biological effectiveness (RBE) of the α-particles used could be estimated from the tumour induction data and found to be 3.8. Mutations in the p53 gene were also observed in these cell lines [16].

Human mammary epithelial cells have proved difficult to transform. Early studies utilised a primary cell line that had been immortalised following treatment with benzopyrene (H185B5). Following exposure of these cells to high linear energy transfer (LET) radiation (2.2 Gy of iron particles), it was possible to select for anchorage-independent growth [17,18]. However, the anchorage-independent cells did not form tumours in thymic nude mice. No detectable rearrangements or deletions in myc, H-rash, Rb, and p53 genes were observed. Some encouraging results were reported using a primary cell strain (MEC 76N) following fractionated doses of gamma irradiation (15×2 Gy). Morphological transformation and development of tumours were observed when the mammary gland area of thymic nude mice was injected [19]. The transformed cells completely lacked p53 function due to a deletion of one allele and a 26-bp deletion in the second allele [20].

Human cell lines immortalised using telomerase

Primary cell cultures of human cells usually require optimal culture conditions to maintain these cells. However, somatic cells exhibit a gradual shortening of the telomeres at each successive division until (eventually) cells undergo senescence after 40–60 cell doublings. Thus, it has proved impossible to undertake transformation studies on these primary cultures. Immortalisation of these primary strains allows cell lines to be developed, but these have a number of disadvantages as various viral constructs or chemical carcinogens are used and these compromise various growth regulatory pathways in the cell.

An alternative approach to immortalising human cells has been utilised recently by transfecting somatic cells with a vector expressing hTERT (the catalytic subunit of telomerase). This approach has markedly extended the life span of these transfected cells [21,22]. Telomerase expression alone does not appear to induce the changes associated with a malignant phenotype [23,24].

A human retinal pigment epithelial cell line (340RPE-T53 hTERT) was exposed to fractionated doses of gamma-irradiation. The cloning efficiency of the cells was measured in soft agar. The parent cell line, like other human epithelial cells, produced only a few clusters under these anchorage-growth independent conditions. The cloning efficiency of the irradiated cells increased markedly in soft agar. Cloned cell lines grown up from individual colonies also demonstrated increased anchorage-independent growth. These irradiated cloned cell lines were also tumourigenic in thymic nude mice whereas the parent cell line did not form tumours. The parent cell line retained a stable diploid karyotype while the irradiated clones exhibited specific chromosome loss and also complex karyotype.

Thus, the study of human cell populations in vitro has developed rapidly. In the field of radiation carcinogenesis, the key step was developing suitable methods enabling somatic cell populations to be immortalised, thereby enabling sufficient cell proliferation to occur before senescence, thus allowing expression of the malignant phenotype. Initially this was achieved using transection of viral constructs. More recently a physiological mechanism (exploited by stem cells to retain their self renewal capacity) has been used by transfecting telomerase into somatic cells thereby providing immortalised cells. In theory, the ultimate aim would be to maintain the key target cells, the stem cells, in vitro and, thus, follow the multi step process from the initiated cell to frank malignancy.

42

Acknowledgements

We would like to thank Dr Andrea Bodnar at Geron Corporation for supplying the cells and the EC Nuclear Fission Safety Program, Nuclear Electric and Scottish Nuclear for financial support.

References

1. Borek C. X-ray induced in vitro neoplastic transformation of human diploid cells. Nature 1980; 283:776−778.
2. Namba M, Nishitani K, Hyodoh F, Fukushima F, Kimoto T. Neoplastic transformation of human diploid fibroblasts (KMST-6) by treatment with ^{60}Co gamma-rays. Int J Can 1985;35: 275−280.
3. Little JB, Su LN, Kano Y. Transformation of human diploid fibroblasts by radiation and oncogenes. In: Rhim JS, Dritschillo A (eds) Neoplastic Transformation in Human Cell Culture: Mechanisms of Carcinogenesis. Totawa, New Jersey: Humana Press, 1991;67−79.
4. O'Reilly S, Walicka M, Kohler SK, Dunstan R, Maher VM, McCormick JJ. Dose-dependent transformation of cells of human fibroblast cell strain MSU-1.1 by cobalt 60 gamma radiation and characterization of the transformed cells. Radiat Res 1998;150:577−584.
5. Redpath JL, Sun C, Colman M, Stanbridge EJ. Neoplastic transformation of human hybrid cells by irradiation. A quantitative assay. Radiat Res 1987;110:468−472.
6. Mendonca MS, Howard K, Fasching CL, Farrington DL, Desmond LA, Stanbridge EJ, Redpath JL. Loss of suppressor loci on chromosome 11 and 14 may be required for radiation induced neoplastic transformation of HeLa × skin fibroblast human cell hybrids. Radiat Res 1998;149:246−255.
7. Thraves P, Salehi Z, Dritschillo A, Rhim JS. Neoplastic transformation of immortalized human epidermal keratinocytes by ionizing radiation. PNAS 1990;87:1174−1177.
8. Rhim JS, Yoo JH, Park JH, Thraves P, Salehi Z, Dritschilo A. Evidence for the multistep nature of in vitro human epithelial cell carcinogenesis. Cancer Res 1990;50:5653−5657.
9. Thraves PJ, Varghese S, Jung M, Grdina DJ, Rhim JS, Dritschilo A. Transformation of human epidermal keratinocytes with fission neutrons. Carcinogenesis 1994;15:2867−2873.
10. Pazzaglia S, Chen XR, Aamodt CB, Wu SQ, Kao C, Gilchrist KW, Oyasu K, Reznikoff CA, Ritter MA. In vitro radiation-induced neoplastic progression of low-grade urothelial tumours. Radiat Res 1994;138:86−92.
11. Hei TK, Piao CQ, Willey JC, Thomas S, Hall EJ. Malignant transformation of human bronchial epithelial cells by radon simulated α-particles. Carcinogenesis 1994;15:431−437.
12. Willey JC, Hei TK, Piao CQ, Madrid L, Willey JJ, Apostolakos MJ, Hukku B. Radiation-induced deletion of chromosomal regions containing tumor suppressor genes in human bronchial epithelial cells. Carcinogenesis 1993;14:1181−1188.
13. Kuettel MR, Thraves PJ, Jung M, Varghese SP, Prasad SC, Rhim JS, Dritschilo A. Radiation-induced neoplastic transformation of human prostate epithelial cells. Cancer Res 1996;56: 5−10.
14. Riches AC, Herceg Z, Bryant PE, Wynford-Thomas D. Radiation-induced transformation of SV40-immortalized human thyroid epithelial cells by single and fractionated exposure to γ-irradiation in vitro. Int J Radiat Biol 1994;66:757−765.
15. Riches AC, Herceg Z, Bryant PE, Stevens DL, Goodhead DT. Radiation-induced transformation of SV40-immortalized human thyroid epithelial cells by single exposure to plutonium α-particles in vitro. Int J Radiat Biol 1997;72:515−521.
16. Gamble SC, Cook MC, Riches AC, Herceg Z, Bryant P, Arrand JE. p53 mutations in tumours derived from irradiated human thyroid epithelial cells. Mutat Res 1999;425:231−238.

17. Yang TC, Stampfer MR, Rhim JS. Neoplastic transformation of human epithelial cells by ionizing radiation. In: Rhim JS, Dritschillo A (eds) Neoplastic Transformation in Human Cell Culture: Mechanisms of Carcinogenesis. Totawa, New Jersey: Humana Press, 1991;103—111.

18. Yang TC, Georgy KA, Tavakoli A, Craise LM, Durante M. Radiogenic transformation of human mammary epithelial cells in vitro. Radiat Oncol Invest 1996;3:412—219.

19. Wazer DE, Chu Q, Liu XL, Gao Q, Safall H, Band V. Loss of p53 protein during radiation transformation of primary human mammary epithelial cells. Molec Cell Biol 1994;14: 2468—2478.

20. Wazer DE, Band V. Molecular mechanisms of immortalisation of human mammary epithelial cells. Radiat Oncol Invest 1996;3:430—434.

21. Bodnar AG, Quellette M, Frolkis M, Holt SE, Chiu CP, Morin GB, Harley CB, Shay JW, Lichtsteiner S, Wright WE. Extension of the life span by introduction of telomerase into normal human cells. Science 1998;279:349—352.

22. Kiyono T, Foster SA, Koo JI, McDougall JK, Galloway DA, Klingelhutz AJ. Both Rb/p16^{INK4a} inactivation and telomerase activity are required to immortalise human epithelial cells. Nature 1998;396:84—88.

23. Jiang XR, Jimenez G, Chang E, Frolkis M, Kusler B, Sage M, Beeche M, Bodnar AG, Wahl GM, Tlsty TD, Chiu CP. Telomerase expression in human somatic cells does not induce changes associated with a transformed phenotype. Nature Genetics 1999;21:111—114.

24. Morales CP, Holt SE, Quellette M, Kaur KJ, Yan Y, Wilson KS, White MA, Wright WE, Shay JW. Absence of cancer-associated changes in human fibroblasts immortalized with telomerase. Nature Genet 1999:21;115—118.

Apoptosis, cell death, and signal transduction

Time-course of apoptosis induction in mouse spleen and thymus after whole-body X-irradiation with fractionated low doses

Kazuko Fujita[1], Takeshi Oda[1], Kazuo Sakai[1], Yoshihiko Akasaka[2], Harumi Ohyama[3] and Takeshi Yamada[1,3]

[1]Komae-Branch, Bio-Science Department, Central Research Institute of Electric Power Industry, Komae-shi, Tokyo; [2]Department of Pathology, Toho University School of Medicine, Ota-ku, Tokyo; and [3]Division of Radiobiology and Biodosimetry, National Institute of Radiological Sciences, Inage-ku, Chiba, Japan

Abstract. Augmentation of immune responses induced by low-dose radiation has been recognized as an example of "radiation hormesis", but the underlying mechanism is still unknown. In this study, we examined the time-course of apoptosis induction by low-dose radiation in the lymphatic organs (aiming to clarify the relationship between the immune augmentation and apoptotic change). After exposure of AKR mice to moderate (4 Gy) or low (0.5 Gy) doses of X-rays, which were given either as a single or a fractionated dose (10 × 0.05 Gy/day), apoptosis in the thymus and spleen was examined using the quantitative in situ end-labeling method. A single dose, whether low or moderate, induced a sharp but transient peak of apoptosis in both organs at 4 h after irradiation. The fractionated exposure caused a biphasic induction of apoptosis in the spleen, but not in the thymus (with the first phase at 6 h and the second 7 days after the last exposure).

Keywords: altruistic cell death, biphasic apoptotic response, radiation hormesis.

Background

Enhancement of the immune response by low-dose radiation is a well known example of radiation hormesis [1]. The proliferative response to mitogenic stimulation by splenocytes can be augmented by exposing mice to whole-body, chronic, intermittent low-dose ionizing radiation [2,3]. However, the mechanism responsible for the hormetic phenomenon is still unknown. Among possible mechanisms, a picture is emerging of the role of apoptosis in the immune organs as an altruistic cell death leading to stimulation of the proliferation of healthy cells.

Apoptosis is relevant to a wide range of biological processes including the immunologic function [4] together with cell injury induced by radiation [5,6]. The induction of extensive apoptosis by injurious stimuli may, in some cases, be explained teleologically by regarding the death as a homeostatic mechanism leading to the selective deletion of cells (whose survival would prejudice the welfare of the host). Thus, it can be argued that apoptosis of cells with significant, unrepaired damage represents altruistic cell suicide [7].

Address for correspondence: Dr K. Fujita, Komae-Branch, Bio-Science Department, Central Research Institute of Electric Power Industry, 2-11-1 Iwado-kita, Komae-shi, Tokyo 201-8511, Japan. Tel.: +81-3-3480-2111. Fax: +81-3-3480-3539. E-mail: abfujita@criepi.denken.or.jp

As yet, however, there is no direct evidence supporting the occurrence of apoptosis in lymphatic organs of mice after exposure to low-dose radiation, and few detailed studies which have dealt with apoptosis in lymphoid organs (in response to very low dose radiation) relevant to the proliferation-augmenting effect. This study examined the detailed time course of apoptosis induction in the spleen and thymus after whole-body (acute or fractionated) low-dose X-irradiation using the in situ histochemical method [8].

Materials and Methods

Animals

AKR/Jsea female mice were used throughout the experiment [8,9]. The experiments using animals were carried out following the Guidelines for the Care and Use of Laboratory Animals established by Ministry of Education, Science, Sport and Culture, Japan.

X-ray irradiation and histological preparations

Whole body X-irradiation as well as histological analyses were performed as described previously [8,9]. Briefly, mice were irradiated using a Hitachi X-ray machine operated at 150 kVp. Two series of the X-ray exposure experiment were performed. In the first series, the total dose of 0.5 Gy was given as a single exposure. In the second, the exposure was given in 10 fractions, namely, each fractionated exposure (0.05 Gy/day) for 5 consecutive days per week, for 2 weeks. The thymus and spleen were removed at various times after irradiation, and each organ was divided into two parts: one for the histological analyses, and the other for the flow cytometric assay.

Histological analyses and flow cytometry

Conventional hematoxylin-eosin (HE) staining, terminal deoxynucleotidyl transferase mediated dUTP-biotin nick-end labeling (TUNEL) [10] and in situ end labeling (ISEL) [11] were performed as previously described [8,9]. Flow cytometric analysis of thymocyte preparation was carried out as previously described [8].

Results

Comparison of the detection sensitivity of the four methods: ISEL, TUNEL, HE staining and flow cytometry

First we compared the above four methods in order to choose the most sensitive and reliable method available for detection of the subtle changes in apoptotic cell number in the lymphoid tissues (following low-dose irradiation). The results

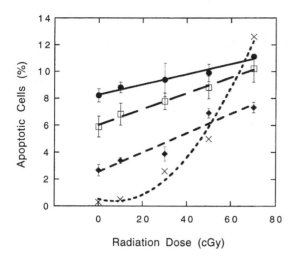

Fig. 1. Comparison of the four detection methods for apoptotic cells in X-irradiated mouse thymus. To compare the detecting sensitivity of the methods, simultaneous assay by ISEL (□), TUNEL (●), HE stain (◆), and flow cytometry (×) was performed using the same thymus 4 h after irradiation with various radiation doses (10–70 cGy) shown on the abscissa. The percentage of apoptotic cells obtained by each method was plotted against the radiation dose.

are shown in Fig. 1. Flow cytometric assay could not detect any apoptotic cells in the low-dose irradiated sample (lower than 20 cGy). HE staining showed the lowest sensitivity. This may have resulted from difficulty in the recognization of early stage apoptotic cells by this method. TUNEL method had the highest sensitivity, but less responsiveness to incremental increases of radiation dose. ISEL method showed sensitivity (almost) comparable to TUNEL and possessed better response to incremental increase in radiation.

Thus we concluded that the ISEL stain was the most suitable method with which to measure apoptosis in low frequency as observed after low-dose irradiation of mice. The ISEL method was used throughout the following experiments for the detection and counting of apoptotic cells. Typical examples of ISEL preparation are shown in Fig. 2.

The apoptotic cells in both the thymus and spleen gradually increased in number immediately following irradiation, then rose sharply to reach the peak level at 4 h regardless of the radiation dose (0.5 or 4 Gy). Thereafter, the apoptotic percent fell rapidly (hour 6) and had returned to normal levels by hour 20. It is of interest to note that the time course of apoptotic change is identical in pattern for both (0.5 and 4 Gy) irradiated groups (data not shown).

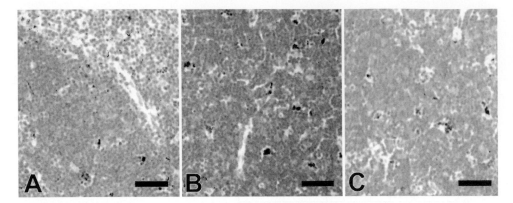

Fig. 2. Thymus 3 (**A**), 4 (**B**) and 5 h (**C**) after 4 Gy whole-body X-irradiation, viewed by the ISEL method. Apoptotic cells are distinct from the surrounding normal cells by their brown color. Bars represent 100 μm.

Biphasic induction of apoptosis in the spleen after fractionated exposure of mice to 0.5 Gy

Stimulative effects of the fractionated low-dose exposure on the splenocyte proliferation reported by Makinodan et al. [2,3] led us to investigate the effects of the fractionated low dose on the splenocyte apoptosis in mice. By dividing 0.5 Gy into 10 equal fractions (a daily exposure of 0.05 Gy, for 5 consecutive days in a week, for 2 weeks), and by extending the observation period to 3 weeks; the second peak of apoptosis was found at day 7 (Fig. 3A) in addition to the first peak

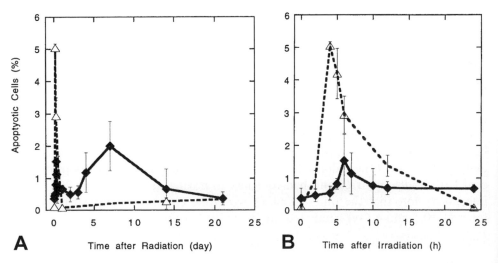

Fig. 3. Time course of apoptosis induction in spleen after a single or fractionated exposure of mice to the total 0.5 Gy X-rays. **A:** Data for 3 weeks. **B:** Replotted data for 24 h. Open triangles with a broken line represent the single exposure, and closed squares with a solid line the fractionated exposure.

a few hours after the last exposure (observed with a single exposure) as described above.

By replotting the data in Fig. 3A, Fig. 3B was obtained, this presented another interesting finding, namely, that the position of the first peak had shifted, appearing not at 4, but at 6 h after the last exposure.

These results indicate that the fractionated low-dose exposure could induce a biphasic apoptotic response in spleen, the first low peak at 6 h and the second high peak 7 days after the last exposure. A single low dose yielded only the highest value, sharp peak at 4 h without the second wave. The biphasic response against the fractionated exposure to low doses was found only with the spleen, but not with the thymus (data not shown).

In this context, it is of interest to note the histological change in the spleen 1 week after exposure (Fig. 4). The difference in histology, especially in the shape and size of the white pulp of the spleen, is apparent between nonirradiated and irradiated mice. The white pulps were decreased in size but increased in number by the fractionated irradiation.

This study shows, for the first time (in the spleen), that fractionated whole-body exposure to low-dose radiation could induce an apoptotic response distinct in time course from the apoptotic change induced by an acute single exposure. Although we have no current ideas as to explaining this phenomenon, these results strongly encourage us to investigate the possibility that apoptosis may play a role in the low-dose induced augmentation of the immune response. Indeed, Shankar et al. [12] recently reported the contribution of apoptosis and p53 to the low-dose induced immunomodulation in C57BL mice. This topic is, accordingly, under current investigation.

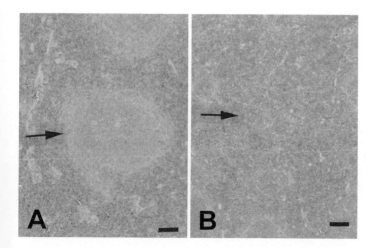

Fig. 4. HE-stained section of the spleen 1 week after 0.5 Gy fractionated whole-body X-irradiation. **A:** Preparation from a nonirradiated control mouse. **B:** Preparation from the irradiated mouse. A typical white pulp is indicated by the arrow. Bars represent 100 μm.

Conclusion

The TUNEL method showed the highest sensitivity among the four apoptosis-detection methods examined. However, the ISEL method showed a sensitivity similar to the nick-end labeling method and a better response to incremental increases of radiation dose.

Single doses, whether low or moderate, induced a sharp but transient peak of apoptosis 4 h after irradiation in both the thymus and the spleen.

The fractionated exposure caused a biphasic induction of apoptosis in spleen, the first peak at 6 h, and the second 7 days after the last exposure. However, the second peak was absent in the thymus.

References

1. Luckey TD. Radiation Hormesis. Boca Raton: CRC Press, 1990.
2. Makinodan T, James SJ. T cell potentiation by low dose ionizing radiation: possible mechanisms. Health Phys 1990;59:29—34.
3. James SJ, Enger SM, Peterson WJ, Makinodan T. Immune potentiation after fractionated exposure to very low doses of ionizing radiation and/or caloric restriction in autoimmune-prone and normal C57BL/6 mice. Clin Immunol Immunopathol 1990;55:427—437.
4. Kerr JFR, Wyllie AH, Currie AR. Apoptosis: a basic biological phenomenon with wide-ranging implications in tissue kinetics. Br J Cancer 1972;26:239—257.
5. Yamada T, Ohyama H. Radiation-induced interphase death of rat thymocytes is internally programmed (apoptosis). Int J Radiat Biol 1988;53:65—75.
6. Ohyama H, Yamada T. Radiation-induced apoptosis: a review. In: Yamada T, Hashimoto Y (eds) Apoptosis, its Roles and Mechanisms. Tokyo: Business Center for Academic Societies Japan, 1998;141—186.
7. Kondo S. Altruistic cell suicide in relation to radiation hormesis. Int J Radiat Biol, 1988;53: 95—102.
8. Fujita K, Ohyama H, Yamada T. Quantitative comparison of in situ methods for detecting apoptosis induced by X-ray irradiation in mouse thymus. Histochem J 1997;29:823—830.
9. Fujita K, Ohtomi M, Ohyama H, Yamada T. Biphasic induction of apoptosis in the spleen after fractionated exposure of mice to very low doses of ionizing radiation. In: Yamada T, Hashimoto Y (eds) Apoptosis, its Roles and Mechanisms. Tokyo: Business Center for Academic Societies Japan, 1998;201—218.
10. Gavriell Y, Sherman YS, Ben-Sasson S. Identification of programmed cell death in situ via specific labeling of nuclear DNA fragmentation. J Cell Biol 1992;119:493—501.
11. Wijsman JH, Jonker RR, Keijzer R, Van de Velde CJH, Cornelisse CJ, Van Dierendonck JH. A new method to detect apoptosis in paraffin sections: in situ end-labeling of fragmented DNA. J Histochem Cytochem 1993;41:7—12.
12. Shankar B, Premachandran S, Bharambe SD, Sundaresan P, Sainis KB. Modification of immune response by low dose ionizing radiation: role of apoptosis. Immunol Lett 1999;68: 237—245.

Effects of low-dose preirradiation on radiation-induced cell death in cultured mammalian cells

Kazuo Sakai

Department of Bio-Science, Central Research Institute of Electric Power Industry, Tokyo, Japan

Abstract. The effects of low-dose preirradiation on the process of radiation-induced cell death were investigated in human embryonic fibroblasts (HE22), and human T cell lymphoma cells (MOLT-4). Analysis of cell growth and the timing of dead cell appearance after irradiation revealed that the process of cell death in HE22 was of mitotic death and that in MOLT-4 was of interphase death. When 10 cGy "conditioning" dose was given 4 h prior to 300 cGy of "challenging" dose, the cell death process was slowed down in HE22, while accelerated in MOLT-4. These results suggested that the effect of preirradiation with small dose of ionizing radiation could differ depending on the type of cells and, presumably, on the type of cell death.

Keywords: adaptive response, apoptosis, dye exclusion test, low-dose radiation.

Background

One of the most well-known effects of low-dose ionizing radiation on the cell is the radiation adaptive response. The adaptive response is defined as the acquired radioresistance after irradiation with low doses, typically 5—20 cGy, of ionizing radiation [1—4]. The underlying mechanisms proposed include the induction of DNA repair mechanisms and the induction of antioxidant substances [5—8]. In addition, modulation of cell death, e.g., inhibition of apoptosis, might be involved in the adaptive response.

To examine the possible involvement of a modification of the cell death process in the adaptive response, we investigated the effect of low-dose ionizing radiation on the dying process in two kinds of cells. The two types of cells showed different types of cell death, mitotic death or interphase death (apoptosis) after irradiation.

Materials and Methods

Cells

Human embryonic fibroblasts, HE22, were kindly supplied by Dr M. Watanabe, Nagasaki University. The cells were cultured in MEM medium supplemented with 10 % fetal calf serum. MOLT-4 cells, human T cells of lymphoma origin,

Address for correspondence: Kazuo Sakai PhD, Bio-Science Department, Central Research Institute of Electric Power Industry, 2-11-1 Iwado-kita, Komae-shi, Tokyo 201-8511, Japan. Tel.: +81-3 3480-2111 (ext. 3356). Fax: +81-3-3480-3539. E-mail: kazsakai@criepi.denken.or.jp

were cultured in RPMI1640 medium supplemented with 10% fetal calf serum. Both were kept at 37°C in a humidified atmosphere containing 5 % CO_2.

Irradiation

The cells were irradiated with X-rays from an X-ray machine (Hitachi) operated at 150 kV (5 mA). The filter used were 0.2 mm Cu and 1mm Al. The irradiation was carried out at room temperature. The dose rate was 0.2 Gy/min.

Dye exclusion test

The cell suspension of MOLT-4 or trypsinized cell suspension of HE22 was mixed with an equal amount of 0.4% erythrosine B in phosphate-buffered saline. The viability of the cells was calculated as the percentage of nonstained cells to the total number of cells examined [9].

Results

Type of cell death in HE22 and MOLT-4

After exposure to 300 cGy of X-rays the cell death process of HE22 was slow; the decrease in viability was not observed until 80 h after irradiation (Fig. 1). The dying process in MOLT-4 was fast; dead cells appeared as early as 10 h after the

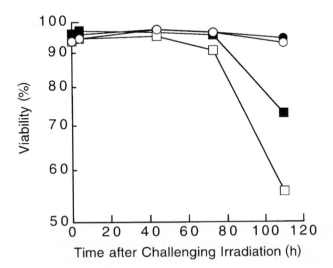

Fig. 1. Effect of preirradiation on the cell death process in HE22. The viability of HE22 cells exposed to 0 cGy (○), 10 cGy (●), 300 cGy (□) only, or 300 cGy of challenging dose 4 h after 10 cGy of conditioning irradiation (■) was analyzed by the dye exclusion test after various periods of postirradiation incubation time.

irradiation (Fig. 2). HE22 continued to grow after the irradiation, while MOT-4 did not show any increase in number (data not shown). These results indicate that the cell death process of HE22 was mitotic death and that of MOLT-4 of interphase death.

Effects of low-dose preirradiation on the cell death process

Irradiation with 10 cGy of a "conditioning" dose 4 h prior to 300 cGy of "challenging" dose slowed down the cell death process in HE22 (Fig. 1). In MOLT-4, on the other hand, the conditioning dose accelerated the process of cell death after the challenging irradiation (Fig. 2). The effects of the low-dose preirradiation were completely opposite between HE22 and MOLT-4. Many reports have shown an increased resistance after the conditioning exposure in various type of cells as in shown here in HE22 [10—13]. Recently, however, the sensitizing effect of preirradiation was reported in terms of the induction of apoptosis in human lymphocytes [14]. As MOLT-4 died an apoptotic death after irradiation [15], we decided to further characterize this "reverse adaptive response".

Dose of conditioning irradiation and the reverse adaptive response

When cells were exposed to various conditioning doses, the acceleration of the cell death was obvious as low as After 5 cGy without any significant cell death by the conditioning dose alone (Fig. 3).

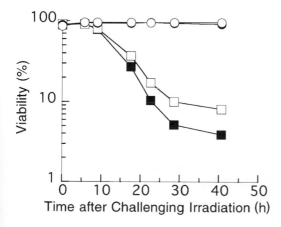

Fig. 2. Effect of preirradiation on the cell death process in MOLT-4. The viability of MOLT-4 cells exposed to 0 cGy (○), 10 cGy (●), 300 cGy (□) only, or 300 cGy of challenging dose 4 h after 10 cGy of conditioning irradiation (■) was analyzed by the dye exclusion test after various periods of postirradiation incubation time.

56

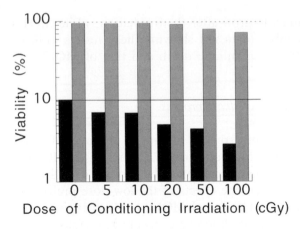

Fig. 3. Dose of the conditioning exposure and the reverse adaptive response. MOLT-4 cells were exposed to 0 to 100 cGy of conditioning dose, followed, 4 h later, by 300 cGy of challenging dose. The viability was analyzed 40 hr after the challenging irradiation. For each dose the gray column indicates the viability of cells exposed to the conditioning dose only, the black column shows that of cells given both the conditioning and the challenging dose. The horizontal solid line and the dotted line in the figure show the level of viability of nonirradiated cells and that of the cells exposed to 300 cGy only.

Interval time and the reverse adaptive response

When the cells were irradiated with 10 cGy, followed by 300 cGy challenging dose after various intervals, and the viability was analyzed 40 h after the challenging irradiation, the viability showed fluctuation with changing length of the interval. Although there was little significance, the interval of 4–6 h seemed to give the most effective acceleration (Fig. 4). This result suggests that some inducible mechanisms, which stimulate the process of apoptosis, might be involved in the reverse adaptive response.

Conclusion

A low priming dose of X-irradiation slowed down the cell death process in HE22 human embryonic fibroblasts, which showed mitotic death after irradiation. The low priming dose of irradiation, on the other hand, accelerated the dying process of MOLT-4 cells, which would die of interphase death.

The effect of low-dose irradiation would be different depending on the type of the cells (or on the type of death) and the time interval between the low and challenge dose.

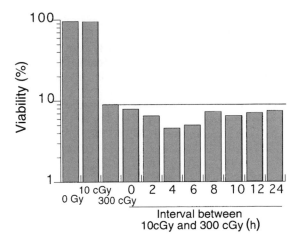

Fig. 4. Interval between the conditioning and the challenging radiation and the reverse adaptive response. MOLT-4 cells pre-exposed to 10 cGy were incubated for various periods and then irradiated with 300 cGy of the challenging dose. The viability of the cells were analyzed 40 h after the challenging irradiation. The three columns to the left in the figure indicate the viability of the cells exposed to 0, 10, or 300 cGy only. The horizontal line in the panel shows the level of the viability of the cells exposed to 300 cGy only.

References

1. Olivieri G, Bodycote J, Wolff S. Adaptive response of human lymphocytes to low concentrations of radioactive thymidine. Science 1984;223,594—597.
2. Seong J, Suh CO, Kim GE. Adaptive response to ionizing radiation-induced by low doses of gamma rays in human cell lines. Int J Radiat Oncol Biol Phys 1995;33:869—874.
3. Shadley JD, Wolff S. Very low doses of X-rays can cause human lymphocytes to become less susceptible to ionizing radiation. Mutagenesis 1987;2:95—96.
4. Shadley JD, Dai G. Cytogenetic and survival adaptive responses in G_1 phase human lymphocytes. Mutat Res 1992;265:273—281.
5. Le XC, Xing JZ, Lee J, Leadon SA, Weinfeld M. Inducible repair of thymine glycol detected by an ultrasensitive assay for DNA damage. Science 1998;280:1066—1068.
6. Ikushima T. Radio-adaptive response: involvement of induction of specific gene expression by low doses of ionizing radiation. In: Sugihara T, Sagan LA, Aoyama T (eds) Low-dose Irradiation and Biological Defense Mechanisms. Amsterdam: Elsevier Science, 1992;255—258.
7. McWilliams RS, Cross WG, Kaplan JG, Birnboim HC. Rapid rejoining of DNA strand breaks in resting human lymphocytes after irradiation by low doses of [60]Co γ-rays or 14.6-MeV neutrons. Radiat Res 1983;94:499—507.
8. Mitchel REJ. Mechanisms of the adaptive response in irradiated mammalian cells. Radiat Res 1995;141:117—118.
9. Sakai K, Suzuki N, Itoh H, Kubodera A. Effects of an inhibitor of protein kinase on the response to heat treatment in cultured mammalian cells. Int J Hyperthermia 1997;13:535—545.
10. Azzam EI, Raaphorst GP, Mitchel REJ. Radiation-induced adaptive response for protection against micronucleus formation and neoplastic transformation in C3H 10T1/2 mouse embryo cells. Radiat Res 1994;138(Suppl):28—31.
11. Birnboim HC, Jevcak JJ. Fluorimetric method for rapid detection of DNA strand breaks in human white blood cells produced by low doses of radiation. Cancer Res 1981;41:1889—1892.

12. Farooqi Z, Kesavan PC. Low-dose radiation induced adaptive response in bone cells of mice. Mutat Res 1993;302:83—89.
13. Kelsey KT, Memisoglu A, Frankel D, Liber HL. Human lymphocytes exposed to low doses of X-rays are less susceptible to radiation-induced mutagenesis. Mutat Res 1991;263:197—201.
14. Cregan SP, Brown DL, Mitchel REJ. Apoptosis and the adaptive response in human lympho-cytes. Int J Radiat Biol 1999;75:1087—1094.
15. Nakano H, Shinohara K. X-ray induced cell death: apoptosis and necrosis. Radiat Res 1994; 140:1—9.

Different radiation-induced response of p53 and WAF1 accumulation after chronic or acute radiation

Akihisa Takahashi, Ken Ohnishi and Takeo Ohnishi

Department of Biology, Nara Medical University, Nara, Japan

Abstract. *Background.* The *p53* gene plays important roles in cancer suppression through induction of cell-growth arrest, DNA repair, or cell death. The *p53* gene regulates expression of downstream genes including *WAF1*, an inhibitor of cyclin-dependent kinase. In this study, we examined whether accumulation of p53 and WAF1 was induced after chronic or acute irradiation.

Methods. Western blot analysis of p53 and WAF1 was applied in cultured human glioblastoma cells after chronic γ-irradiation (0.001 Gy/min) or acute X-irradiation (1.33 Gy/min).

Results. Acute irradiation at 3 Gy induced accumulation of p53 and WAF1. After chronic irradiation of 3 Gy for 50 h, a challenge of acute irradiation (at 0.3 or 1.0 Gy) did not have any further efficacy in inducing accumulation of these proteins (even if accumulation was observed during chronic irradiation). However, the challenge of acute irradiation 48 h after cessation of chronic irradiation induced accumulation of these proteins.

Conclusions. These findings indicate that chronic irradiation at a low dose rate induced accumulation of p53 and WAF1 in a different manner from that after acute irradiation. This suggests that chronic irradiation at a low dose rate may induce a different signaling pathway (for radiation response) from that induced after acute irradiation.

Keywords: cultured human cells, low dose rate, recovery of response, signal transduction.

Introduction

Modulation of gene expression in response to ionizing radiation is of prime interest in the field of radiation biology. In most articles concerning biological responses to ionizing radiation, it has been found that radiation-induced gene expression (after irradiation in the lethal dose range, 2–50 Gy) has been reported. The biological effect of low-dose radiation on cellular responses has received recent attention because protection against low-dose radiation (less than 1 Gy) may be required as a factor of life. Although epidemiological data regarding the cancer incidence from areas with high background radiation levels seems to favor a beneficial effect of chronic low-dose radiation [1–3], the molecular mechanisms remain unclear. It has been considered that p53 is not only a guardian of the genome but also an integrator of stress-response signals [4,5]. The *p53* gene exerts various biological functions through transactivation of downstream genes including *WAF1* [6]. The *p53* gene plays important roles in

Address for correspondence: Takeo Ohnishi, Department of Biology, Nara Medical University, 840 Shijo-cho Kashihara-shi, Nara 634-8521, Japan. Tel.: +81-744-22-3051 (ext. 2264). Fax: +81-744-25-3345. E-mail: tohnishi@nmu-gw.naramed-u.ac.jp maintaining genomic stability as a cell cycle checkpoint in G_1 and G_2/M transition [6—8] and an effector of DNA repair [9,10] or apoptosis [11,12]. We previously reported that p53 accumulation was induced in several organs of whole-body irradiated mice and rats (receiving less than 0.5 Gy [13,14]), and that pre-irradiation of the cells with chronic γ-rays (at a low dose rate) blunted the response of p53 and WAF1 to a challenge of acute irradiation in cultured human glioblastoma cells [15].

In this study, we analyzed the cellular content of p53 and WAF1 after various schedules of irradiation (in cultured human glioblastoma cells) in order to examine whether chronic irradiation at a low dose rate induces WAF1 expression in a different manner from acute irradiation.

Materials and Methods

Cell culture

Human glioblastoma A-172 cells (provided by JCRB, Setagaya, Tokyo, Japan) bearing the wild-type *p53* gene are competent in activating the expression of a p53-regulated gene such as *WAF1*. These cells were cultured in DMEM containing 10% (v/v) fetal bovine serum, penicillin (50 U/ml), streptomycin (50 μg/ml) and kanamycin (50 μg/ml).

Irradiation procedure

Chronic γ-irradiation (0.001 Gy/min) was administered with a ^{137}Cs γ-source (Sangyo Kagaku Co., Ltd., Tokyo, Japan) located in the Radiation Research Center, Kyoto University, Japan. Chronic γ-irradiation was delivered to cells cultured at 37°C in an incubator. Acute X-irradiation (1.33 Gy/min) was administered with a Radioflex 350 (250 kV, 15 mA at room temperature) X-ray source (Rigaku, Tokyo, Japan).

Western blot analysis

Cells were washed with phosphate-buffered saline (PBS), centrifuged and pelleted at 4°C. The cells were resuspended in RIPA buffer (50 mM Tris, pH 7.2, 150 mM NaCl, 1% (v/v) NP-40, 1% (w/v) sodium deoxycholate and 0.05% (w/v) sodium dodecylsulfate (SDS)), and then exposed to three cycles of freezing and thawing. The protein content of the supernatants obtained after centrifugation (10,000 g, 15 min) were quantified using a BIO-RAD Protein Assay Kit (Bio Rad Laboratories, California, USA). Protein (20 μg per lane) was loaded on 10 or 15% (w/v) polyacrylamide gels containing 0.1% (w/v) SDS and underwent electrophoretic transfer onto polyvinylidene difluoride membranes, the proteins on each membrane were incubated with an antihuman p53 monoclonal antibody (DO-1) and an antihuman WAF1 monoclonal antibody (EA10) (Oncogene

Science Inc., New York, USA). The bands were visualized using a horseradish peroxidase-conjugated goat antimouse IgG antibody (Zymed Laboratories Inc., California, USA) and the blotting amplification system (BLAST) (DuPont/ NEN Research Products, Massachusetts). The amounts of p53 and WAF1 in samples were calculated (relative to those in controls) by scanning the profiles of the bands obtained using the public domain NIH Image program (written by Wayne Rasband at the US National Institutes of Health). The details about Western blot analysis are described elsewhere [16].

Results

In order to clarify the radiation response of p53 and WAF1 against acute challenge irradiation, we applied Western blot analysis (for p53 and WAF1) in cultured human glioblastoma cells after irradiation with chronic γ- (0.001 Gy/min) or acute X-irradiation (1.33 Gy/min).

Dose-dependence of p53 and WAF1 accumulation after acute irradiation in A-172

Initially, we determined the dose-dependence of p53 and WAF1 accumulation following acute radiation (Fig. 1A). The amounts of p53 and WAF1 were measured after 1.5 and 6 h, respectively. As shown in Fig. 1A, the p53 level increased 2.6-, 3.0-, and 3.7-fold by 0.3, 1.0, and 3.0 Gy, respectively, at a dose-rate of 1.33 Gy/min (compared with that in the nonirradiated control). WAF1 accumulation showed a pattern similar to that of p53, increasing 2.2-, 3.8-, and 4.4-fold after 0.3, 1.0, and 3.0 Gy irradiation (again, compared with the WAF1 level in the nonirradiated control). A linear dose-dependent response in the range of 0.3–1.0 Gy was observed at this high dose rate (Fig. 1A).

Time-course dependence of p53 and WAF1 accumulation

Regarding p53 accumulation, chronic and acute irradiation produced a biphasic response (Fig. 1B,C). During chronic irradiation, the first p53 peak appeared at 1.5 h (0.09 Gy) and the second peak at 10 h (0.54 Gy). However, WAF1 expression exhibited a single peak at 10 h and declined gradually thereafter. It was notable that the p53 level was even lower than that of the basal level after 24 h (1.44 Gy) or 50 h (3.0 Gy) (Fig. 1B). After 3 Gy of acute irradiation alone, p53 accumulated as early as 1.5 h after exposure, while accumulation of WAF1 reached a maximum 6 h after exposure (Fig. 1C).

Accumulation of p53 and WAF1 by challenge irradiation

When acute irradiation was performed on cells exposed to chronic γ-rays for 50 h (3 Gy), accumulation of p53 and WAF1 was not induced in these cells (Fig. 1D). In the case of acute preirradiation (3.0 Gy) however, p53 and WAF1 accu-

62

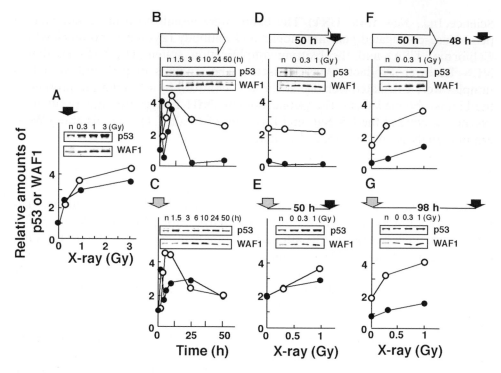

Fig. 1. p53 and WAF1 inducibility by chronic (0.001 Gy/min) or acute (1.33 Gy/min) irradiation in A-172 cells. Chronic irradiation represented by a hollow arrow right, 3 Gy of acute irradiation by a shaded arrow down, various doses of acute irradiation by a solid arrow down. "n" represents non-irradiated control samples; ●, the relative amounts of p53; and ○, the relative amounts of WAF1. **A:** Dose-dependence of p53 and WAF1 accumulation, after acute irradiation. The amounts of p53 and WAF1 were measured at 1.5 and 6 h, respectively. **B:** Time-course dependence of p53 and WAF1 accumulation during chronic irradiation. **C:** Time-course dependence of p53 and WAF1 accumulation after 3 Gy of acute irradiation. Accumulation of p53 and WAF1 following various doses of the second acute challenge irradiation. **D:** Accumulation immediately after chronic irradiation (50 h, 3 Gy). **E:** Accumulation 50 h after 3 Gy of acute irradiation. **F:** Accumulation 48 h after chronic irradiation (50 h, 3 Gy). **G:** Accumulation 98 h after 3 Gy of acute irradiation. The amounts of p53 and WAF1 were measured at 1.5 and 6 h (respectively) after challenge irradiation.

mulation (following the second acute challenge irradiation) was observed 50 h after preirradiation (Fig. 1E). The accumulation of p53 and WAF1 in response to the acute challenge irradiation was observed 48 h after cessation of chronic preirradiation (50 h at 3.0 Gy) (Fig. 1F), as is the case with acute X-ray pre-irradiation at 3.0 Gy (Fig. 1E,G).

Discussion

The intracellular ratio of mutated p53 to wild-type p53 increased under normal culturing conditions and was unchanged after radiation [17]. Using Western blot analysis, it could not be detected whether p53 was the active, or inactive form (even when p53 accumulated after the addition of cellular stress). However, *WAF1* gene expression is directly regulated by p53 through the p53 binding activity (at the transcriptional level) to the specific consensus sequence located upstream of the *WAF1* gene [6]. Therefore, the detection of WAF1 induction is useful for the analysis of p53-mediated signal-transducing activity in cells exposed to stress. Thus, we measured the amounts of p53 and WAF1 using Western blot analysis.

Our study found that chronic preirradiation with γ-rays at a low dose rate for 50 h (total dose of 3.0 Gy) could attenuate the p53-dependent response to an acute postirradiation in cultured human glioblastoma cells (Fig. 1D). On the contrary, acute preirradiation at 3.0 Gy did not affect the p53-dependent response to acute postirradiation 50 h after the preirradiation (Fig. 1E). This different p53 response to acute irradiation may be due to different preirradiation conditions. When p53-dependent signal transduction was constantly activated, p53 could not respond to the challenge irradiation. Indeed, we found that the responsiveness of the p53-dependent signal transduction, as measured by accumulation of p53 and WAF1 to acute postirradiation, could recover 48 h after the cessation of chronic preirradiation (Fig. 1F). These findings support our assumption that attenuation of p53 and WAF1 accumulation, in response to acute postirradiation by chronic preirradiation, is transient. In other words, the nonresponsive period of p53 induction after chronic preirradiation is severely limited. It is clear that the responsiveness of radiation-induced signal transduction is dependent on environment during signaling.

This raises an important question about the mechanism that induces non-responsiveness of p53 after chronic irradiation at a low dose rate; we consider three possible mechanisms: 1) lack of emergency signals to induce DNA repair and/or to reduce DNA damage induced by chronic irradiation; 2) perturbation of signaling in response to radiation; and 3) loss of response to control cell cycle. The lack of emergency signals may be supported by findings relating the adaptive response to damage reduction by the induction of radical detoxification and/or repair systems [18]. However, perturbation of signaling may be supported by the fact that low-dose radiation activates protein kinase C (PKC) shortly after exposure to ionizing radiation [19,20]. The observation that inhibitors of PKC completely block the adaptive response supports the hypothesis that the transduction of the low dose-induced signal involves PKC activation [20,21]. Recently, it has been reported that PKC upregulates the binding activity of p53 to p53CON by phosphorylating serine 378 at the carboxyl terminal domain of p53 [22]. We have previously reported that the binding activity of p53 to p53CON was inhibited by a specific PKC inhibitor [23]. These results, including our findings, suggest that suppression of PKC activity by chronic irradiation may cause downregulation of *WAF1* gene expression. Some other steps in p53 phosphorylation by the phosphatidylinositol 3-kinase family (including ATM and DNA-dependent kinase) may be necessary for p53 activation in those cells [24,25]. The third possibility: loss

64

of response to regulate cell cycle, may be supported by the report that chronically irradiated cells were synchronized at a nonresponsive stage in their cycle so that *WAF1* gene expression was not induced [26]. However, it remains unclear what induces the nonresponsiveness of cells to acute irradiation challenge after chronic irradiation. In addition, another question is raised about how chronic radiation compromises the p53-dependent response which controls gene stability. The end-points of p53 response are decreased mutation and chromosomal aberration [27—29]. Based on present observations, we consider that this phenomenon may be due to the wearing away of the p53-dependent response by chronic irradiation at a low dose rate. If this is verified, it will further strengthen the notion of p53 as "the Guardian of the Genome" [4], thus recognizing that chronic irradiation at low doses may have harmful effects on health (such as cancer induction) by compromising p53, an idea which is (apparently) still lacking substantial support at present. Further evidence from studies of p53-dependent endpoints (such as apoptosis) may facilitate a better understanding of the role of p53 responses depressed by chronic irradiation at a low dose rate [30]. Finally, we suggest that elucidation of the effects of chronic irradiation (at a low dose rate) is a highly important issue in radiation biology regarding human health.

Acknowledgements

This work was partly supported by the Japan Atomic Energy Research Institute under contract to the Nuclear Safety Research Association and the Central Research Institute of Electric Power Industry in Japan. This study was also funded in part by "Ground Research for Space Utilization" promoted by NASDA and Japan Space Forum.

References

1. Sugahara T. Radiation paradigm and its shift. J Radiat Res 1994;35:48—52.
2. Wang Z, Boice JD, Wei L, Beebe GW, Zha Y, Kaplan MM, Tao Z, Maxon HR III, Zhang S, Schneider AB, Tan B, Wesseler T, Chen AD, Ershow AG, Kleinerman RA, Littlefield LG, Preston D. Thyroid nodularity and chromosome aberrations among women in area of high background radiation in China. J Natl Cancer Inst 1990;82:478—485.
3. Mifune M, Sobue T, Arimoto H, Komoto Y, Kondo S, Tanooka H. Cancer mortality survey in a spa area (Misasa, Japan) with a high radon background. Jpn J Cancer Res 1992;83:1—5.
4. Lane D. p53, guardian of the genome. Nature 1992;358:15—16.
5. Wang X, Ohnishi T. p53-dependent signal transduction induced by stress. Radiat Res 1997;38: 179—194.
6. El-Deiry WS, Tokino T, Velculescu VE, Levy DB, Parsons R, Trent JM, Lin D, Mercer WE, Kinzler KW, Vogelstein B. WAF1, a potential mediator of p53 tumor suppression. Cell 1993;75: 817—825.
7. Dulic V, Kaufman W, Wilson S, Tisty T, Lees E, Harper J, Elledge S, Reed S. p53-dependent inhibition of cyclin-dependent kinase activities in human fibroblasts during radiation-induced G_1 arrest. Cell 1994;76:1013—1023.
8. Agarwal ML, Agarwal A, Taylor WR, Stark GR. p53 controls both the G_2/M and the cell cycle

checkpoints and mediates reversible growth arrest in human fibroblasts. Proc Natl Acad Sci USA 1995;92:8493—8497.

9. Kastan M, Zhan Q, El-Deiry WS, Carrier F, Jacks T, Walsh W, Plunkett B, Vogelstein B, Fornance A Jr. A mammalian cell cycle checkpoint pathway utilizing p53 and GADD45 is defective in ataxia-telangiectasia. Cell 1992;71:587—597.

10. Mummenbrauer T, Janus F, Muller B, Wiesmuller L, Deppert W, Grosse F. p53 protein exhibits 3'-to-5' exonuclease activity. Cell 1996;85:1089—1099.

11. Miyashita T, Reed JC. Tumor suppressor p53 is a direct transcriptional activator of the human *bax* gene. Cell 1995;80:293—299.

12. Caelles C, Helmberg A, Karin M. p53-dependent apoptosis in the absence of transcriptional activation of p53-target genes. Nature 1994;370:220—223.

13. Wang X, Matsumoto H, Okaichi K, Ohnishi T. p53 accumulation in various organs of rats after whole-body exposure to low-dose X-ray irradiation. Anticancer Res 1996;16:1671—1674.

14. Wang X, Matsumoto H, Takahashi A, Nakano T, Okaichi K, Ihara M, Ohnishi T. p53 accumulation in the organs of low-dose X-ray irradiated mice. Cancer Lett 1996;104:79—84.

15. Ohnishi T, Wang X, Takahashi A, Ohnishi K, Ejima Y. Low dose rate radiation attenuates the response of the tumor suppressor TP53. Radiat Res 1999;151:368—372.

16. Wang X, Takahashi A, Ohnishi K, Matsumoto H, Suda K, Ohnishi T. Bifunctional effects of a protein kinase inhibitor (H-7) on heat-induced p53-dependent WAF1 accumulation. Exp Cell Res 1997;237:186—191.

17. Oren M, Maltzman W, Levine AJ. Post-translational regulation of the 54K cellular tumor antigen in normal and transformed cells. Molec Cell Biol 1981;1:101—110.

18. Rigaud O, Moustacchi E. Radioadaptation for gene mutation and the possible molecular mechanisms of the adaptive response. Mutat Res 1996;358:127—134.

19. Woloschack GE, Chang-Liu C, Jones PS, Jones CA. Modulation of gene expression in syrian hamster embryo cells. Cancer Res 1990;50:339—344.

20. Liu SZ. Multilevel mechanisms of stimulatory effect of low-dose radiation on immunity. In: Sugahara T, Sagan LA, Aoyama T (eds) Low-Dose Irradiation and Biological Defense Mechanisms. Amsterdam: Elsevier, 1992;225—232.

21. Ikushima T. Radio-adaptive response: involvement of specific genes induction by low doses of ionizing radiation. In: Sugahara T, Sagan LA, Aoyama T (eds) Low-Dose Irradiation and Biological Defense Mechanisms. Amsterdam: Elsevier, 1992;255—258.

22. Takenaka I, Morin F, Seizinger BR, Kley N. Regulation of the sequence-specific DNA binding function of p53 by protein kinase C and protein phosphatases. J Biol Chem 1995;270:5405—5411.

23. Ohnishi K, Wang X, Takahashi A, Ohnishi T. Contribution of protein kinase C to p53-dependent WAF1 induction pathway after heat treatment in human glioblastoma cell lines. Exp Cell Res 1998;238:399—406.

24. Canman CE, Lim DS, Cimprich KA, Taya Y, Tamai K, Sakaguchi K, Appella E, Kastan MB, Siliciano JD. Activation of the ATM kinase by ionizing radiation and phosphorylation of p53. Science 1998;281:1677—1679.

25. Woo RA, Malure KG, Lees-Miller SP, Rancourt DE, Lee PW. DNA-dependent protein kinase acts upstream of p53 in response to DNA damage. Nature 1998;394:700—704.

26. Marin LA, Smith CE, Langston MY, Quashie D, Dillehay LE. Response of glioblastoma cell lines to low dose rate irradiation. Int J Radiat Oncol Biol Phys 1991;21:397—402.

27. Yamagishi N, Miyakoshi J, Takebe H. Decrease in the frequency of X-ray induced mutation by wild-type p53 protein in human osteosarcoma cells. Carcinogenesis 1997;18:695—700.

28. Schwartz JL, Russell KJ. The effect of functional inactivation of TP53 by HPV-E6 transformation on the induction of chromosome aberrations by gamma rays in human tumor cells. Radiat Res 1999;151:385—390.

29. Bouffler SD, Kemp CJ, Balmain A, Cox R. Spontaneous and ionizing radiation-induced chromosomal abnormalities in p53-deficient mice. Cancer Res 1995;55:3883—3889.

66

30. Sasaki MS. Radioadaptive response: an implication for the biological consequences of low dose rate exposure to radiations. Mutat Res 1996;358:207—213.

The effects of small doses of radiation on intestinal stem cells

Christopher S. Potten and Dawn Booth

Epithelial Biology Department, Paterson Institute for Cancer Research, Christie Hospital NHS Trust, Manchester, UK

Abstract. Small doses of radiation (< 1 Gy) kill the actual lineage ancestor stem cells (ASC) in the crypts of the small intestine but not in the large intestine. The sensitivity of these stem cells suggests that this might be a protective mechanism for removing cells carrying DNA damage, thus reducing the risk for cancer development in the small bowel. Here we have investigated the effects of small priming doses of radiation (that kill a proportion of these ASC) on the survival of the potential clonogenic regenerative stem cells (PSC) in the crypt using the crypt microcolony assay. The PSC are greater in number and possess a higher radioresistance, possibly as a consequence of higher levels of expression of the p53 protein. Priming doses of radiation tend to render the PSC compartment slightly more resistant in the small bowel, but more sensitive in the large intestine. There are suggestions that the extrapolation number (which is related to the number of PSC in the crypt) is reduced at the time when the maximum apoptotic death occurs at 4 h, this number is further reduced at 2 days, the time when the apoptotic susceptible ASC are replaced. These effects are accentuated following high priming doses of radiation.

Keywords: apoptosis, crypt microcolonies intestine, low-dose irradiation, stem cells.

The epithelium lining the gastrointestinal tract has been extensively studied in relation to its proliferation kinetics, the cellular lineages, and the radiobiological response. The epithelium in the small intestine and large intestine (of the mouse) is well characterised, and represents a highly polarised, simple columnar epithelium, one cell thick, with well defined proliferative units (the crypts) providing cells for the differentiated functional part of the tissue. This, in the small intestine, is organised into discrete units called villi, and in the large intestine is simplified to a differentiated intercrypt table epithelium. The continual loss of worn out functional cells into the lumen of the intestine is compensated precisely by cell division in the crypts [1]. Cell production in the crypts is organised within discrete cell lineages. Each crypt in the small and large intestine of the mouse is believed to contain about four to six such lineages and hence four to six lineage ancestor stem cells (ASC) [2]. These self-maintaining stem cells produce daughters that enter a dividing transit population which is characterised by about six generations in the small intestine and up to eight generations in the large intestine [3]. Consideration of a wide range of cell kinetic and radiobiological studies have suggested that the commitment to differentiation (i.e., loss from the stem

---

Address for correspondence: Christopher S. Potten, Epithelial Biology Department, Paterson Institute for Cancer Research, Christie Hospital NHS Trust, Wilmslow Road, Manchester M20 4BX, UK. Tel.: +44-161-446-3125. Fax: +44-161-446-3181. E-mail: cpotten@picr.man.ac.uk

cell compartment) is in fact not made until a cell is two or three generations down the lineage [3]. Under steady state conditions of cell replacement, these uncommitted potential stem cells (PSC) inexorably move through the cell generations, undergoing differentiation at a specific point, while continuing to divide for the prescribed number of generations, before becoming mature functional differentiated cells that migrate onto the villus and intercrypt table. However, under experimental laboratory conditions the actual or ancestral stem cells (ASC) can be killed by, for example, low doses of radiation, in which case cells from the potential stem cell compartment can repopulate the ASC compartment, the full cell lineage and, hence, ultimately parts of the entire epithelium. This is achieved through a process of clonal cell divisions, and the production of clones that can be recognised histologically. This forms the basis of the crypt microcolony assay that has been extensively studied and interpreted [4,5].

Unfortunately, as yet, there are no stem cell specific markers that enable either the ASC or PSC to be marked (and hence identified) in tissue sections. However, the highly polarised intestinal epithelium has the great advantage of having the cell lineages oriented along the long axis of the crypt. As a consequence, the position that the ASC and PSC occupy in the crypt can be identified, hence the cells that occur at these positions can be studied. In the small intestine the critical position is immediately above the functional differentiated Paneth cells, i.e., at about cell position 4 from the crypt base. In particular regions of the large intestine there is an absence of any cells equivalent to Paneth cells, thus the stem cell location is right at the crypt base.

Using detailed cell positional analysis in both cell kinetic, immunohistochemical, histology, and radiobiological experiments, we have identified a number of features associated with the stem cell position. These include:

1. A slower cell cycle at cell position 4 in the small intestine than for the majority of the transit cells [6].
2. Cell lineage tracking studies in the small and large bowel indicate that the origin of all cell migration occurs at cell position 4 in the small intestine, and 1 in the large intestine [7].
3. There is strong expression of wild-type p53 protein in some cells at the stem cell position following exposure to cytotoxic agents (including radiation) [8].
4. There is expression of bcl-2 protein in the stem cell position in the large bowel, but not in the small intestine [9].
5. A high propensity for apoptosis to be induced in a p53-dependent manner at the stem cell position in the small intestine following low doses of radiation [8,10,11].

This high susceptibility for apoptosis induction of some cells at the stem cell position in the small intestine has been interpreted as a protective mechanism whereby cells that incur DNA damage altruistically commit suicide, thus removing the damage and the cell [12,13]. This process does not occur in the large intestinal stem cells due to the expression of the survival gene bcl-2 [9]. This process has been suggested as part of the explanation for the rarity of cancer development in the small intestine, a tissue with an inherently high cell proliferation (cellular turnover), and large tissue mass, both of which might suggest high levels of cancer risk, whereas, the contrary is actually observed [12].

Thus, one of the most obvious effects of exposure of the intestinal epithelium to small doses of radiation is the rapid induction of apoptosis in the stem cell region of the small intestinal crypts. These cells exhibit an extremely high radiosensitivity, with the dose-response data indicating significant elevations in the level of apoptosis following 5 cGy, and detectable changes following doses as low as 1 cGy [10,11,14]. This apoptosis is p53 dependent (being absent in p53 knockout mice) [8]. However, the apoptotic cells do not appear to express immunohistochemically detectable levels of wild-type p53 protein. High levels of p53 protein are however, detectable in adjacent nonapoptotic cells at the stem cell location interpreted to be the PSC population. The apoptosis appears rapidly with peak values being observed within 3 to 6 h, the peak yield being centered on cell position 4 (Fig. 1), and the dose-response data indicating that all the susceptible cells are killed by doses between 0.5 and 1 Gy (and, that at this level of exposure the crypt contains about 6 apoptosis susceptible cells at cell position 4) (Fig. 1). Once saturation levels have been reached for apoptosis induction, i.e., when all 6 susceptible cells have been killed, the crypts all survive and are presumed to be regenerated from other potential stem cells. Once regeneration is complete

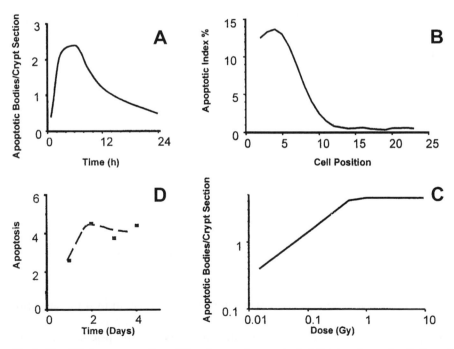

Fig. 1. Simplified representation of the changes in apoptosis following dose of radiation. **A:** Time-course following 0.22 Gy. **B:** Cell position following 0.63 Gy. **C:** Re-establishment of the apoptosis susceptible population at various times following 0.5 Gy [15]. **D:** Dose response on a log/log scale.

the apoptosis susceptible population is re-established. In fact the apoptosis susceptible cells can be detected about 2 days after radiation [15] (Fig. 1). If the doses of radiation are increased further into the range 9—16 Gy, progressively more of the PSC per crypt are reproductively sterilised by these increasing doses. These reproductively sterilised cells do not, in the most part, die via apoptosis but are presumed to prematurely differentiate and hence persist in the tissue as functional cells ultimately displaced onto the villus. If one or more of the potential stem cells survive in the crypt, it is capable of regenerating the entire crypt lineage and the crypt structure within a period of about 3 days. This forms the basis of the crypt microcolony assay, where surviving regenerated crypts are counted between days 3 and 4 postirradiation [4,5]. The data generated in this way can be used to estimate the number of cells per crypt that possess crypt regeneration capacity, i.e., the number of potential clonogenic stem cells. The obtained estimates for the number of PSC depends somewhat on the levels of stress (radiation exposure or DNA damage) that are imposed upon the crypt. At the lowest level of stress (i.e., low radiation doses of less than 9 Gy), the data suggest 6 PSC per crypt, i.e., the immediate non-ASC daughters of the ASC population. In other words the first generation down the lineage. At high levels of stress (doses greater than 9 Gy), the data suggest that up to about 30 cells per crypt may be capable of being triggered to function as PSC, i.e., numbers consistent with the second and (part of the) third generation down the lineage [16]. This leaves about 120 other proliferating cells that have apparently lost all potential to function as stem cells. Studies in aged mice suggest that this restriction to the second or third generation is relaxed in old mice and, as a consequence, many more cells (each of which might have poorer quality DNA) may be recruited into the PSC compartment [17].

We have recently undertaken a series of experiments designed to see if the effects of killing the apoptosis-susceptible ASC influence the radiosensitivity of the clonogenic potential stem cells (and hence the shape of the crypt survival curve in the microcolony assay). The studies have been undertaken by delivering a small priming dose of radiation (at various times) before a series of graded large doses. The priming dose was generally 0.5 Gy and the microcolony assay test doses ranged between and 10 and 16 Gy. Microcolonies were assessed between days 4 and 5 postirradiation. The small priming dose of radiation was delivered either:

1. Four hours before the large dose, i.e., a time interval equivalent to the time of peak apoptotic yield.
2. One day before the large dose, i.e., a time significant for the removal of the apoptotic cells, but before the full re-establishment of the apoptotic susceptible cells.
3. Two days before the large dose, i.e., a time equivalent to the point of re-establishment of the apoptotic susceptible population.
4. Four days before the large dose, i.e., a time equivalent to the assay time for the microcolony assay.

5. Seven days before the large dose, i.e., a time equivalent to the full re-establishment of the intestinal integrity (a time in excess of the intestinal turnover
   time).

In some experiments both the small intestine and colon have been studied. For
the small intestine the crypt microcolony assay was performed on day 4, and
for the midcolon region, the microcolony assay was scored on day 5. In a few
cases smaller or larger priming doses were used. The counts have been corrected
for size variations in the colonies in each experiment [18].

The data are presented as a series of crypt survival curves (with crypt survival
plotted on a logarithmic scale against dose on a linear scale). These curves char-
acteristically have a large shoulder, an area of curvature and an exponential relationship between crypt survival and dose (as the last remaining clonogenic cell
is reproductively sterilised as dose increases). The shoulder region is interpreted
as being the consequence of the product of the number of clonogenic cells per
crypt and the repair capacity for each clonogenic cell. The curves are defined by
the D_0 value, which is the mean lethal dose (a measure of clonogenic cell radiosensitivity), and the extrapolation number N (which is the value obtained by
extrapolating the linear exponential region of the dose response curve back to
zero dose). N is thus a measure of the size of the shoulder and is mainly attributable to the product of the number of PSC per crypt and the individual cell repair
capacity of the PSC.

Since the experiments were designed to investigate whether the effects of a
small priming dose influenced the shape of a subsequent crypt survival curve,
the data have been plotted using only the final large dose of radiation and not
the sum of the priming dose plus the final dose.

To determine the number of surviving crypts, 10 transverse sections were
counted for the number of surviving crypts per circumference (a convenient unit
of length) and a minimum of four mice per dose was used. The individual mean
value for each mouse was entered into the DRFIT programme which fitted
curves, determined the D_0 and N values with their confidence intervals, and
undertook statistical comparisons between one survival curve and the next [18].

Figure 1A shows a typical set of data for apoptotic yield vs. time for a small
dose of radiation where peak yields are observed between 3 and 6 h. Also shown
is a typical cell positional distribution obtained at the time of the peak yield for
the small intestine, with maximum numbers of apoptotic bodies being observed
around the fourth and fifth position in the crypt (Figure 1B). A typical curve for
the increasing yield of apoptoses with increasing radiation dose is shown in Fig.
1C. Figure 1D shows data summarising the experiments of Ijiri and Potten [15],
indicating that the apoptotic susceptible cell population is re-established about
2 days after a priming dose of radiation.

The results of the survival curves are summarised in Tables 1 and 2 and Figs.
2—6, where the dosing schedule is shown together with the number of animals
used to generate the crypt survival curve in each case (numbers in parenthesis),
as well as the parameters that define the curves (D_0, the N value, and the dose

Table 1. Analysis of small intestine crypt survival curves.

Treatment	D_0 (Gy)	N	D50 (Gy)	p
All control groups (72)	1.415	836.4	10.04	—
0.25 Gy 4 h (24)	1.522	442.3	9.83	0.1737
0.25 Gy 2 days (24)	1.518	563.3	10.17	0.0448
0.5 Gy wait 4 h (48)	1.491	433.9	9.60	<0.001
0.5 Gy wait 6 h (24)	1.526	507.8	10.07	0.2141
0.5 Gy wait 1 day (24)	1.473	494.3	9.68	0.2956
0.5 Gy wait 2 days (24)	1.758	155.1	9.52	0.2966
0.5 Gy wait 4 Days (24)	1.515	488.1	9.93	0.4176
0.5 Gy wait 7 Days (24)	1.460	583.2	9.83	0.9828
0.1 Gy 4 h (24)	1.485	561.6	9.95	0.7079
0.1 Gy 2 days (24)	1.489	759.1	10.00	<0.001
0.1 Gy 4 days (24)	1.426	931.8	10.27	0.0126
2.5 Gy wait 4 h (24)	2.213	40.6	9.02	<0.001
2.5 Gy wait 2 days (30)	1.915	127.1	9.99	<0.001
5 Gy 4 h (24)	3.066	6.0	6.78	<0.001
5 Gy 2 days (30)	2.306	42.1	9.49	<0.001

required to reduce crypt survival to 50% (D50 dose)) and the p value for the comparison between the survival curve and the control survival curve (i.e., the crypt survival curve obtained using no priming dose). There was no significant difference between the survival curves obtained at different times after a priming dose of 0.5 Gy (Table 1 and Fig. 2), however, the data obtained for the 2-day split showed a reduction in the N value, the overall curves, however, were not significantly different (p = 0.0966). This trend of a reduction in N value for the small intestine was seen in all the experiments involving different priming doses given 2 days before the full test doses. The curves were significantly different at 2 days, when the priming dose was 1 Gy for the small intestine (p<0.001) (see Fig. 4). Interestingly, for the midcolon, although the clonogenic cells here are more resistant (the curves have a higher Do and a lower value of N), all the survival curves with the exception of those for the 7 day interval were statistically significantly different from the control curve, largely due to a reduction in the D50. Figure 2

Table 2. Analysis of colon crypt survival curves.

Treatment	D_0 (Gy)	N	D50 (Gy)	p
All control groups (23)	2.675	69.41	12.34	—
0.5 Gy wait 4 h (24)	2.524	70.68	11.69	0.0176
0.5 GY wait 1 day (24)	2.523	57.62	11.17	<0.001
0.5 Gy wait 2 days (23)	2.659	51.21	11.46	0.0019
0.5 Gy wait 4 days (24)	2.530	58.37	11.23	<0.001
0.5 Gy wait 7 days (24)	3.025	36.62	12.03	0.2293

Number of mice in parenthesis; p values for comparison of entire survival curve

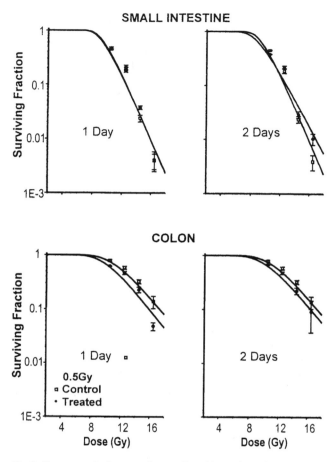

SMALL INTESTINE

COLON

1 Day

2 Days

1 Day

0.5Gy
▫ Control
• Treated

2 Days

Fig. 2. Crypt survival curves for small and large intestine generated 1 and 2 days after 0.5 Gy priming dose.

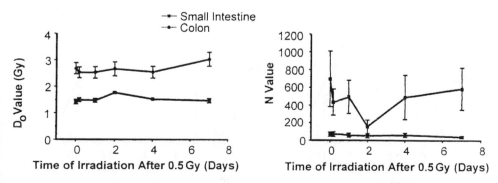

Fig. 3. D_0 and N values for survival curves obtained at various times after a priming dose of 0.5 Gy.

74

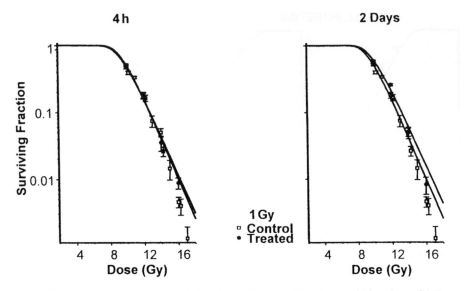

Fig. 4. Crypt survival curves generated at 4 h and 2 days, following a priming dose of 1 Gy.

shows representative crypt-survival curves for the small intestine and midcolon for the day 1 and day 2 split data, while Fig. 3 shows the D_0 and N values for the data involving priming doses of 0.5 Gy for the small intestine and colon. The trend of a fall in the N value in the small intestine for the 2-day split is evident. Figures 4–6 show the 4-h and 2-day split survival curves for the 1-, 2.5-, and 5.0-Gy priming doses. For all the curves there is a strong tendency for a reduction

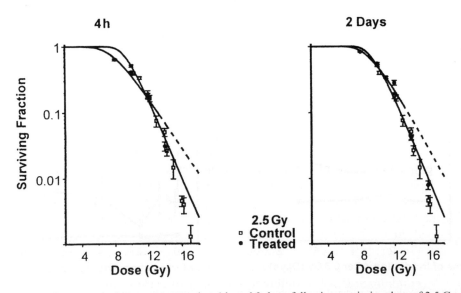

Fig. 5. Crypt survival curves generated at 4 h and 2 days, following a priming dose of 2.5 Gy.

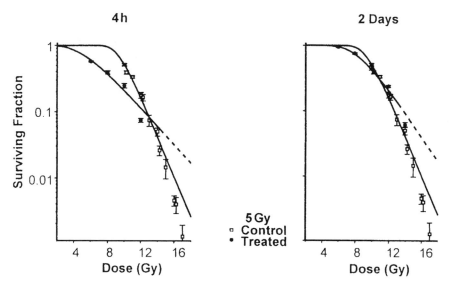

Fig. 6. Crypt survival curves generated at 4 h and 2 days, following a priming dose of 5 Gy.

in the extrapolation number when there is a 4-h split. This becomes significant for doses above 1 Gy, but the trend is also observed at 0.25 and 0.5 Gy. By 2 days after the higher priming doses the shoulder begins to be re-established, while for the lower priming doses the N values seem to show a fall at day 2.

These data can be interpreted on the basis of our current model of an hierarchical stem cell population in the crypt, with six steady state ASC that have a very high radiosensitivity and a larger population of PSC with a high radioresistance. The smaller priming doses cause a reduction in number of the ASC, which the earlier data of Ijiri and Potten suggested are not repopulated until day 2. The present experiments might suggest that this repopulation of killed ASC is achieved at the expense of the clonogenic compartment, i.e., potential clonogenic stem cells assume the mantle of ASC without undergoing any cell division, and as a consequence, the clonogenic compartment is reduced by approximately the number of ASC killed. Since these priming doses would kill most of the ASC in the crypts, estimated to be about six in number, this, in turn, would suggest that the PSC compartment is reduced by about six. As the radiation doses increased beyond about 1 Gy, more of the potential clonogenic cells are reproductively sterilised. This is seen in the data for the 4-h split as a dramatic reduction in the shoulder on the crypt survival curve. By day 2 clonal regeneration has largely re-established the crypt stem cell population, and the shoulder reappears on the crypt survival curve. There is the suggestion that these regenerated clonogenic cells have a greater radioresistance (higher D_0) either as a consequence of the priming effects of the first dose (i.e., making repair phenomena more rapid or efficient) or as a consequence of differences in the cell cycle status of the clonogenic compartment (in a steady state crypt) compared to a regenerated crypt at day 2.

It is interesting that, as would be predicted, subtle differences are observed between the small and large intestine concerning the effects of small sized priming doses. Firstly, there is a slight trend for an increase in the D_0 value for the small intestine data (i.e., a shift to greater resistance for splits of various times up to 2 days following 0.5 Gy, a shift to the right of the survival curves), while in the large intestine for the same split times, and the same priming dose, there is a tendency for a decrease in the D_0 values, i.e., greater sensitivity (a shift to the left in the survival curves). Secondly, the fall in the extrapolation number seen at 2 days for the small intestine, is not observed as dramatically for the large intestine. These differences could be attributable to the fact that, in the small intestine the 6 ASC exhibit a high radiosensitivity and large propensity to undergo apoptosis (a protective mechanism against genetic damage), while in the large intestine the 6 ASC express bcl-2 and, as a consequence, have a greater radioresistance in terms of apoptosis induction. The genetic damage that is induced by the small priming dose may then persist and contribute to the total accumulated damage leading to an increased propensity for reproductive sterility when the high doses are delivered. The data observed here for the small intestine showing a trend towards greater survival levels in the samples that received a small priming dose are consistent with similar trends observed for jejunal crypt cells by others [19].

Acknowledgements

This work was supported by the Cancer Research Campaign and the Central Research Institute for the Electric Power Industry (CRIEPI), Japan.

References

1. Potten CS. Structure, function and proliferative organisation of mammalian gut. In: Potten CS, Hendry JH (eds) Radiation and Gut. Amsterdam: Elsevier, 1995;1–31.
2. Potten CS, Booth C, Pritchard M. The intestinal epithelial stem cell: the mucosal governor. Int J Exp Path 1997;78:219–243.
3. Potten CS. Stem cells in gastrointestinal epithelium: numbers, characteristics and death. Phil Trans R Soc Lond B 1998;353:821–830.
4. Withers HR, Elkind MM. Microcolony survival assay for cells of mouse intestinal mucosa exposed to radiation. Int J Radiat Biol 1970;17:261–268.
5. Potten CS, Hendry JH. The microcolony assay in mouse small intestine. In: Potten CS, Hendry JH (eds) Cell Clones: Manual of Mammalian Cell Techniques. Edinburgh: Churchill Livingston, 1985;50–60.
6. Potten CS. Cell cycles in cell hierarchies. Int J Radiat Biol 1986;49:257–278.
7. Qiu JM, Roberts SA, Potten CS. Cell migration in the small and large bowel of mice shows a strong circadian rhythm. Epith Cell Biol 1995;3:138–150.
8. Merritt AJ, Potten CS, Hickman JA, Kemp C, Balmain A, Hall P, Lane D. The role of p53 paper in spontaneous and radiation-induced intestinal cell apoptosis in normal and p53-deficient mice. Cancer Res 1994;54:614–617.

9. Merritt AJ, Potten CS, Watson AJM, Loh DY, Hickman JA. Differential expression of bcl-2 in intestinal epithelia: correlation with attenuation of apoptosis in colonic crypts and the incidence of colonic neoplasia. J Cell Sci 1995;108:2261—2271.

10. Potten CS. Extreme sensitivity of some intestinal crypt cells to X- and γ- irradiation. Nature 1977;269:518—521.

11. Potten CS, Grant H. The relationship between radiation-induced apoptosis and stem cells in the small and large intestines. Br J Cancer 1998;78:993—1003.

12. Potten CS. The significance of spontaneous and induced apoptosis in the gastrointestinal tract of mice. Cancer Metastasis Rev 1992;11:179—195.

13. Potten CS, Li YQ, O'Connor PJ, Winton DG. Target cells for the cytotoxic effects of carcinogens in the murine large bowel and a possible explanation for the differential cancer incidence in the intestine. Carcinogenesis 1992;13:2305—2312.

14. Hendry JH, Potten CS, Chadwick C, Bianchi M. Cell death (apoptosis) in the mouse small intestine after low doses: effects of dose-rate 14.7 MeV neutrons and 600 MeV (maximum energy) neutrons. Int J Radiat Biol 1982;42:611—620.

15. Ijiri K, Potten CS. The re-establishment of hypersensitive cells in the crypts of irradiated mouse intestine. Int J Radiat Biol 1984;46:609—624.

16. Cai W, Roberts SA, Potten CS. The number of clonogenic cells in three regions of murine large intestinal crypts. Int J Rad Biol 1997;71:573—579.

17. Martin K, Potten CS, Kirkwood TBL. Altered stem cell regeneration in irradiated intestinal crypts of senescent mice. J Cell Sci 1998;111:2297—2303.

18. Potten CS, Rezvani M, Hendry JH, Moore JV, Major D. The correction of intestinal micro-colony counts for variations in size. Int J Radiat Biol 1981;40:321—326.

19. Roberts SA. DRFIT: a programme for fitting radiation survival models. Int J Radiat Biol 1990; 57:1243—1246.

20. Hendry JH. A new derivation, from split-dose data, of the complete survival curve for clono-genic normal cells in vivo. Radiat Res 1979;78:404—414.

Adaptive responses and immune responses

Radioadaptive response: its variability in cultured human lymphocytes

Takaji Ikushima[1] and S.M. Javad Mortazavi[2]

[1]Biology Division, Kyoto University of Education, Kyoto, Japan; [2]Faculty of Medical Sciences, Tarbiat Modares University, Tehran, Iran

Abstract. *Background.* The molecular mechanism behind the radioadaptive response still remains unclear, however, the involvement of inducible DNA repair has been indicated. The generality of the phenomenon has yet to be established since the radioadaptive response has been found to be dependent upon many factors (such as the adapting dose, dose rate, cell cycle, culture conditions, and the genetic constitution of individuals, with some being unresponsive). Here, using peripheral blood lymphocytes from healthy Asian donors, the dependency of the radioadaptive response on X-ray photon energy (within the diagnostic range) was studied, and a follow-up study was also carried out in a nonresponder.

Methods. Cultured lymphocytes were exposed to an adapting dose of 5 or 10 cGy (from 70 to 150 kVp X-rays) at 24 h of culture and subsequently to a challenging dose of 2 or 3 Gy at 48 h.

Results. Three donors responded with reduced incidence of chromatid aberrations in all photon energies, high energy X-rays being most effective, whereas one donor did not respond. The nonresponder did not show the radioadaptive response at any kVp at any time during the period of a 6 month follow-up study.

Conclusion: There is a considerable interindividual variability in human lymphocytes with respect to the adaptation expression.

Keywords: adaptive response, chromatid aberration, interindividual variability, low dose.

Introduction

Radiation biology research this century has created a paradigm, "even the lowest doses are harmful and to be avoided". Recently, however, several new phenomena have been found in cellular responses to low doses of radiation, throwing doubts on this paradigm. Among them, the radioadaptive response may be one of the most interesting and novel phenomena. When cells are exposed to a small dose of ionizing radiation and then to a large dose a few hours later, the latter dose-induced genotoxic effects may be less than if the cells were exposed to the large dose alone.

This adaptive response was first reported by Olivieri et al. [1] for radiation-induced chromosomal aberrations in human lymphocytes. Radioadaptive responses have been repeatedly demonstrated since then not only for the induc-

Address for correspondence: Takaji Ikushima, Biology Division, Kyoto University of Education, 1 Fukakusa-Fujinomori, Fushimi, Kyoto 612-8522, Japan. Tel.: +81-75-644-8266. Fax: +81-75-645-1734. E-mail: ikushima@kyokyo-u.ac.jp

tion of chromosomal aberrations but also for a wide variety of endpoints, such as gene mutation, cell killing, and neoplastic transformation [2—5]. The existence of the radioadaptive response has also been pointed out at the cellular level for somatic and germinal cells in many kinds of eukaryotes (such as human, hamster, mouse, goldfish, and higher plants), suggesting a universal phenomenon. The radioadaptive response may be beneficial to cells with respect to its contribution to the maintenance of genomic integrity. Despite the molecular mechanism behind the radioadaptive response not being elucidated, evidence for a faster and enhanced repair of DNA double-strand breaks in adapted cells has been cleverly obtained using a single-cell gel electrophoresis [6]. The radioadaptive response may be defined as the induction of double-strand break repair by small doses of radiation.

On the other hand, the radioadaptive response (in terms of chromosomal aberrations) has been shown to vary from one donor to another with some individuals being unresponsive and a few exhibiting a synergistic response to the two doses [7,8]. The reasons for this interindividual variability remain unsolved, and the generality of the radioadaptive response has yet to be established. This point may be important, especially in its relevance to radiogenic risk prediction [9]. So, we have investigated the ability of cultured human lymphocytes (from healthy Asian donors) to adapt to different radiation exposures so that the yield of chromosomal aberrations induced by a subsequent exposure is reduced. Furthermore, considering the possible implications of induced radioprotective mechanisms for human health, we have attempted to test whether or not the magnitude of radioadaptive response will change with different X-ray photon energies in the diagnostic range. Here we present new data that indicate an interindividual variability of radioadaptive response in human lymphocytes from Asian donors as well as a long-term follow-up study in a nonresponder, thus considering the generality of radioadaptive response.

Materials and Methods

Venous blood samples were drawn from healthy adult donors of both sexes into heparinized vacutainers. Whole blood (0.7 ml) was added to 10 ml RPMI 1640 medium containing 20% fetal calf serum (Bio Whittaker), 2 mM L-glutamine, 25 mM HEPES, 2.5% PHA-M (GIBCO BRL) and antibiotics. The blood was cultured in 5 ml plastic tissue culture flasks (Falcon) at $37°C$ in a 5% CO_2 atmosphere.

The cells were exposed to the adapting dose of 5 or 10 cGy of X-rays at 0.247 Gy/min, 24 h after PHA stimulation. The challenge dose of 2 or 3 Gy of X-rays was given 48 h after PHA stimulation. All irradiations were carried out with a SOFTEX X-ray machine (M-150WS). Exposures were at 5 mA, 70, 100, 130, and 150 kVps with 0.1 mm Cu + 0.5 mm Al filters. The doses were monitored by LiF thermal luminescence dosimetry.

Fifty-two hours after PHA stimulation, colcemid (final concentration 2×10^{-7} M) was added to all cultures to arrest the dividing lymphocytes in mitosis. At 54 h the cells were harvested, exposed to 0.075 M KCl for 10 min at 37°C, and fixed with methanol acetic acid (3:1 v/v). The fixed cells were dropped onto wet slides, air dried, and stained with Giemsa.

Chromatid-type aberrations were scored in 100 well-spread metaphases with 46 chromosomes for each data point. Gaps or achromatic lesions were not included. The expected number of chromatid aberrations was calculated as follows: expected number = number of aberrations induced by adapting dose + number of aberrations induced by challenge dose – number of aberrations in the unirradiated cells. Student's t test was used to determine the significance of the differences between the observed and expected number of chromatid aberrations.

Results and Discussion

When peripheral blood lymphocytes from healthy donors (two Asian males and two Asian females, aged 22 to 40) were exposed to a 5 cGy of adapting dose (24 h after PHA stimulation) and subsequently to a 2 Gy challenge dose (48 h after stimulation), the radioadaptive response was observed in three donors, but not in one male donor. As shown in Fig. 1, a considerable interindividual variability in radioadaptive response induction was apparent among Asian donors, as has been shown in non-Asian donors [7]. The first, second, and third donors had

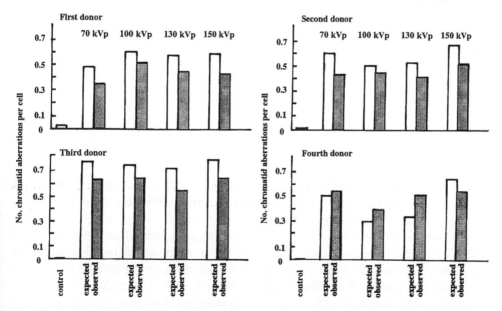

Fig. 1. Frequency of chromatid aberrations induced by an adapting dose of 5 cGy followed by a challenge dose of 2 Gy in lymphocytes from four human donors.

the ability to induce the radioadaptive response by very small doses of X-rays at all four different photon energies (70—150 kVp), its magnitude being lowest in the third donor.

These data are the first to show the adaptive response in peripheral blood lymphocytes from Japanese donors. More efficient induction of the radioadaptive response was observed with 70 kVp and 150 kVp of X-rays. To compare different photon energies of X-rays with regard to the effectiveness of the adaptive response induction, the ratio of the observed frequency of chromatid aberrations to the expected one was calculated using the data averaged over the three donors. These values were 0.758, 0.867, 0.784, and 0.769 for 70, 100, 130, and 150 kVp, respectively. The consistent dependency of the radioadaptive response induction on the radiation quality of X-rays, however, could not be clearly demonstrated within the diagnostic radiology range tested here.

In contrast with these three donors, the fourth donor (male, non-Japanese Asian aged 34) did not show a radioadaptive response at any kVp point (Fig. 1). There was one kVp point where there was a synergistic effect of the two doses on the induction of chromatid aberrations. This nonsmoker nonresponder has no alcohol or drug consumption, and no history of irradiation or viral infection. The lack of radioadaptive response has been previously reported in some individuals, but the cause is not necessarily clear [8]. It has been shown that the presence or absence of a radioadaptive response may be determined by possible transient physiological parameters [8].

To know whether or not the absence of the radioadaptive response in the fourth donor is a temporal situation, the induction of the radioadaptive response was monitored at different times over six months (at intervals of two months). The results of this follow-up study are given in Table 1. In the first experiment, the cells were irradiated with an adapting dose of 10 cGy and then challenged with 3 Gy X-rays. The observed values for chromatid aberrations were higher than the expected values at all of four kVp points. For 130 and 150 kVp, significant synergistic effects were observed.

In the second experiment, there was still a point (70 kVp) with significant synergistic effect ($p < 0.01$), but the differences between observed and expected values for chromatid aberrations were not significant for the other three kVp points.

In the third experiment, the cells were pre-exposed to 5 cGy and challenged with 2 Gy. Again, the cells did not show radioadaptive response at any kVp point, there being a point (130 kVp) with significant synergistic effect. Since the irradiation schemes were identical for the first and second experiment, the results of each kVp point were compared. This comparison suggested some changes in the radiosensitivity for chromosomal aberration induction per se during the period of the follow-up study, but never a higher susceptibility to radiation than in other responders. Nevertheless, the lack of radioadaptive response was observed in each series of experiments with different X-ray qualities. Some reports have showed a nonresponder among patients with chromosome instability syndromes

Table 1. Follow-up study of radioadaptive response induction in a nonresponder.

Treatment	No. chromatid aberrations per cell				
	No radiation	X-ray voltage			
		70 kVp	100 kVp	130 kVp	150 kVp
The first experiment					
Control	0.01				
10 cGy		0.02	0.02	0.02	0.02
3 Gy		0.25	0.39	0.29	0.30
10 cGy + 3 Gy		0.40	0.50	0.64	0.84
(expected value)		(0.26)	(0.41)	(0.30)[b,d]	(0.31)[c,d]
The second experiment					
Control	0.00				
10 cGy		0.03	0.03	0.03	0.03
3 Gy		0.40	0.54	0.45	0.65
10 cGy + 3 Gy		0.66	0.41	0.58	0.52
(expected value)		(0.43)[b,d]	(0.57)	(0.48)	(0.68)
The third experiment					
Control	0.00				
5 cGy		0.03	0.03	0.03	0.03
2 Gy		0.51	0.37	0.34	0.65
5 cGy + 2 Gy		0.54	0.40	0.51	0.54
(expected value)		(0.54)	(0.40)	(0.37)[a,d]	(0.68)

[a]$p < 0.05$; [b]$p < 0.01$; [c]$p < 0.001$; [d]synergistic effect.

such as Down syndrome and ataxia telangiectesia [10,11]. It has also been suggested that ageing might be a factor which abolishes the adaptive response [12]. These findings, however, may not correspond to the lack of the adaptive response of the present nonresponder. The results suggest that the absence of the radioadaptive response is probably not a temporary situation.

Though more experiments are needed to confirm the absence of adaptive response, it may be tentatively concluded that some genetic constitution of each individual plays an important role in determining the presence or absence of the radioadaptive response. Since the study of (the origin of) the absence of radioadaptive response is very important (and helps in elucidating the mechanisms of adaptive response), similar long-term follow-up studies should be performed with a larger number of negative adaptation donors.

Acknowledgements

This work was supported by a fund from the Central Research Institute of Electric Power Industry. The authors wish to thank Y. Ishii and Y. Ejima for their technical assistance.

References

1. Olivieri G, Bodycote J, Wolff S. Adaptive response of human lymphocytes to low concentrations of radioactive thymidine. Science 1984;223:594—597.
2. Ikushima T. Chromosomal response to ionizing radiation reminiscent of an adaptive response in cultured Chinese hamster cells. Mutat Res 1987;80:215—221.
3. Joiner MC. Induced radioresistance: an overview and historical perspective. Int J Radiat Biol 1994;65:79—84.
4. Rigaud O, Papadopoulo D, Moustacchi E. Decreased deletion-type mutation in radioadapted human cells. Radiat Res 1993;133:94—101.
5. Azzam EI, Raaphorst GP, Mitchel REJ. Radiation-induced adaptive response for protection against micronucleus formation and neoplastic transformation in C3H 10T1/2 mouse embryo cells. Radiat Res 1994;138(Suppl):S28—S31.
6. Ikushima T. Radioadaptive response: efficient repair of radiation-induced DNA damage in adapted cells. Mutat Res 1996;358:193—198.
7. Sankaranarayanan K, Von Duyn A, Loos M, Natarajan AT. Adaptive response of human lymphocytes to low level radiation from radioisotopes or X-rays. Mutat Res 1989;211:7—12.
8. Olivieri G, Bosi A. Possible causes of variability of the adaptive response in human lymphocytes. In: Obe G, Natarajan ED (eds) Chromosomal Aberrations: Basic and Applied Aspects. Berlin: Springer-Verlag, 1990;130—139.
9. United Nations Scientific Committee on the Effects of Atomic Radiation (UNSCEAR). Sources and Effects of Ionizing Radiation. New York: United Nations, 1994.
10. Khandogina EK, Mutovin GR, Zvereva SV, Antipov AV, Zverev DO, Akifyev AP. Adaptive response in irradiated human lymphocytes: radiobiological and genetical aspects. Mutat Res 1991;251:181—186.
11. Nemethova G, Kalina I, Racekova N. The adaptive response of peripheral blood lymphocytes to low doses of mutagenic agents in patients with ataxia telangiectasia. Mutat Res 1995;348: 101—104.
12. Gadhia PK. Possible age-dependent adaptive response to a low dose of X-rays in human lymphocytes. Mutagenesis 1998;13:151—152.

The duration of radioadaptive response in mouse bone marrow cells in vivo

Dmitry Yu. Klokov[1], Svetlana I. Zaichkina[1], Olga M. Rozanova[1], Gella F. Aptikaeva[1], Asia Kh. Akhmadieva[1], Elena N. Smirnova[1] and Vladimir Y. Balakin[2]

[1]*Institute of Theoretical and Experimental Biophysics RAS, Pushchino; and* [2]*Branch of the Institute of Nuclear Physics SD RAS, Protvino, Russia*

Abstract. *Background.* Most studies of radioadaptive response have concentrated on in vitro systems. Little experimentation has been done concerning the long-term dynamics of the adaptive response in vivo. The aim of the present study was to investigate the duration of the adaptive response induced by various low doses of γ-radiation in mice in in vivo.

Methods. The frequency of micronucleated polychromatic erythrocytes in mouse bone marrow, determined by means of micronucleus test, was used as a biological end-point.

Results. Doses of 0.1 and 0.2 Gy induced the adaptive response that persisted for up to 8 and 12 months, respectively. In contrast to the above doses, a dose of 0.4 Gy induced the adaptive response for 2 weeks, then disappeared.

Conclusions. The results implicate the role (of the level) of cytogenetic damage per unit dose in inducing short- or long-term adaptive response.

Keywords: adaptive response, in vivo, radiation.

Introduction

Despite extensive studies carried out on entirely different objects (human [1] and rabbit [2] lymphocytes, mouse [3] and rat [4] bone marrow cells, and plant cells [5]) since the first observation by Olivieri et al. [6], the mechanisms underlying adaptive response (AR) are still unclear. Most research has concentrated on in vitro systems, and although there have been a number of in vivo AR studies [7,8], the results obtained have been contradictory [8,9].

Moreover, in most works, AR was only examined for a short period (3–24 h) after irradiation with the adaptive dose (D_1). Only two works have been reported in which AR was studied for prolonged intervals. In one of them, AR was recognized by the mouse bone marrow colony-forming units over a period of 28 days after in vivo low-dose γ-irradiation [3]. The authors of another paper have demonstrated the increased survival of mice after sublethal doses of X-irradiation 2 months after preliminary exposure to low doses [10].

Address for correspondence: Mr Dmitry Yu. Klokov, Institute of Theoretical and Experimental Biophysics, Pushchino, Moscow region 142292, Russia. Tel.: +7-0967-739-349. Fax: +7-0967-790-553. E-mail: dimokl@mail.ru

The aim of the present study was to investigate the duration of the AR induced by various D_1 doses of γ-rays in mouse bone marrow cells in vivo.

Materials and Methods

In our experiments, we used SHK male mice. The animals were kept at a constant temperature and humidity ($23 \pm 3°C$, $50 \pm 5\%$) and housed 10 to a plastic cage with a 12-h dark-light cycle. They were fed nutritional pellets and given water ad libitum. For D_1-dose irradiation, 2-month-old mice were used. The animals were cared for in accordance with the guidelines of the Russian Academy of Sciences for animal care and treatment.

γ-irradiation (^{60}Co) was given as a single whole-body dose. One-half of the animals were irradiated with the D_1 dose (0.1, 0.2 or 0.4 Gy; 0.12 Gy/min). At definite intervals, mice from preirradiated and control groups were irradiated with the challenge dose (D_2) (1,5 Gy; 1 Gy/min). Animals were killed by cervical dislocation 28 h after D_2 dose, and bone marrow slides were prepared using the standard procedure [11]. The number of micronucleated polychromatic erythrocytes (MPCE) were counted. From each mouse, 1,000–2,000 PCE were analyzed. Each experimental point is an average of the experimental data for no less than five mice. For each time interval, the background level of cytogenetic damage was determined; 6,000 PCE from each animal were taken. Statistical analysis was performed using Student's t test.

Results

In the experiments with the D_1 dose of 0.1 Gy, the intervals between irradiations with the D_1 and D_2 doses were 24 h, 2 weeks and 1–12 months (Table 1). At each interval, the levels of cytogenetic damage in the primed (D_1+D_2) animals were lower than those in the unprimed (D_2) group. Figure 1 shows the dynamics of changes in the relative value of AR, which was calculated as the ratio of expected to observed frequency of MPCE. It can be seen from Table 1 that the 0.2 Gy D_1 dose induced the AR at all the time intervals studied (24 h, 2 weeks, 1–8 months). Figure 1 clearly demonstrates that both doses 0.1 and 0.2 Gy are effective in inducing the AR (though the value of the AR induced by the latter is less pronounced). The experiments with the D_1 dose of 0.4 Gy revealed that by month 1 and 2 the AR was absent (Fig. 1), with the maximum AR being registered 24 h after irradiation (Table 1).

Discussion

The present results demonstrate that the 0.1 and 0.2 Gy D_1 doses induced a persistent AR in contrast to the AR induced by the 0.4 Gy D_1 dose (which is absent by months 1 and 2). It is difficult to unambiguously explain this phenomenon, and the literature data (on the effect of the D_1 dose on the dynamics of AR

Table. 1. Frequency of MPCE in bone marrow of mice γ-irradiated in vivo with D_1 and D_2 doses in various modes.

Time between D_1 and D_2	Treatment	Percent[a] of MPCE ± SE[b]		
		For D_1 = 0.1 Gy	For D_1 = 0.2 Gy	For D_1 = 0.4 Gy
24 hours	D_1	0.92 ± 0.16	1.52 ± 0.22	2.29 ± 0.57
	D_2	7.9 ± 0.7	7.7 ± 0.7	7.6 ± 0.7
	D_1+ D_2	4.9 ± 0.7[d]	5.3 ± 0.2[d]	5.1 ± 0.5[e]
2 weeks	D_1	0.50 ± 0.08	0.47 ± 0.04	2.7 ± 0.22
	D_2	5.6 ± 0.4	7.7 ± 0.7	8.3 ± 0.6
	D_1+ D_2	3.0 ± 0.4[e]	5.5 ± 0.2[c]	7.5 ± 0.8[c]*
1 month	D_1	0.14 ± 0.05	0.14 ± 0.06	0.61 ± 0.07
	D_2	7.6 ± 0.5	6.1 ± 0.4	8.7 ± 0.4
	D_1+ D_2	4.2 ± 0.3[d]	4.1 ± 0.4[d]	8.9 ± 0.4
2 months	D_1	0.11 ± 0.05	0.14 ± 0.06	0.60 ± 0.21
	D_2	9.2 ± 1.1	6.5 ± 0.5	6.6 ± 0.4
	D_1+ D_2	5.2 ± 0.4[d]	3.2 ± 0.4[e]	6.4 ± 0.4
3 months	D_1	0.44 ± 0.11	0.13 ± 0.09	
	D_2	8.3 ± 0.6	6.9 ± 0.5	
	D_1+ D_2	5.4 ± 0.8[d]	4.0 ± 0.3[d]	
4 months	D_1	0.44 ± 0.11		
	D_2	8.3 ± 0.6		
	D_1+ D_2	4.7 ± 0.5[d]		
7 months	D_1	0.15 ± 0.12		
	D_2	6.1 ± 0.5		
	D_1+ D_2	4.1 ± 0.5[c]		
8 months	D_1		7.1 ± 0.7	
	D_2		4.4 ± 0.2[d]	
	D_1+ D_2			
9 months	D_1	6.1 ± 0.3		
	D_2	3.9 ± 0.2[d]		
	D_1+ D_2			
12 months	D_1	5.8 ± 0.3		
	D_2	3.7 ± 0.3[d]		
	D_1+ D_2			

[a]The means are given without background level of MPCE frequency; [b]SE is standard error; [c]$p < 0.05$; [d]$p < 0.01$; [e]$p < 0.001$.

induction in vivo) are limited and contradictory [3–7].

Currently several factors have been considered to be involved in the AR induction, including triggering the expression of some genes whose products are thought to be related to DNA repair and control of cell cycle progression [12,13], structural rearrangement of chromatin [14], etc. The precise mechanisms of the AR initiation, however, are still unknown.

Of important note are the 0.1 and 0.2 Gy D_1 doses, as compared to the D_1 dose of 0.4 Gy, which cause an equal level of cytogenetic damage per unit dose in mouse bone marrow in vivo [15]. The dose of 0.4 Gy corresponds to the next

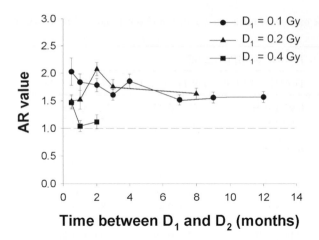

Fig. 1. The dependence of the relative AR value on time between D_1 and D_2 doses. Results of the experiments with the D_1 doses of 0.1, 0.2 and 0.4 Gy are shown.

linear portion of the dose-response curve of in vivo micronucleus induction. Therefore, based on the data presented, it can be assumed that the induction of AR over short and prolonged periods of time is due to two different mechanisms. Furthermore, our results suggest that the involvement of these mechanisms, depends on the value of D_1 doses which induce different initial levels of cytogenetic damage per unit dose.

References

1. Shadley JD. Chromosomal adaptive response in human lymphxocytes. Radiat Res 1994;138 (Suppl):S9—S12.
2. Liu SZ, Cai L, Sun SQ. Induction of cytogenetic adaptive response by exposure of rabbits to very low dose-rate γ-radiation. Int J Radiat Biol 1992;62(2):187—190.
3. Semenets TN, Semina OV, Saenko AS. Phenomenon of adaptive resistance to gamma-irradiation of colony-forming units (CFU-S): manifestation in exogenous test. Radiat Biol Radioecol 1993;33(4):525—528.
4. Klokov DYu, Zaichkina SI, Aptikaeva GF, Akhmadieva AKh, Rozanova OM, Ganassi EE. Induction of cytogenetic damages by combined chronic and acute gamma radiation in rat bone marrow cells. Russ J Genet 1997;37(6):855—857.
5. Cortes F, Mateos JS. Premature onset of mitosis and potentiation of chromosome damage induced by poly-D-lysine in plant cells: evidence for G_2 repair. Mutat Res 1991;247:147—151.
6. Olivieri G, Bodycote J, Wolff S. Adaptive response of human lymphocytes to low concentrations of radioactive thymidine. Science 1984;223:594—597.
7. Yonezawa M, Misonoh J, Hosokawa Y. Two types of X-ray-induced radioresistance in mice: presence of 4 dose ranges with distinct biological effects. Mutat Res 1996;358:237—243.
8. Zhang L. Cytogenetic adaptive response induced by pre-exposure in human lymphocytes and marrow cells of mice. Mutat Res 1995;334:33—37.
9. Wojcik A, Bonk K, Muller WU, Streffer C, Weissenborn U, Obe G. Absence of adaptive response to low doses of X-rays in preimplantation embryos and spleen lymphocytes of an inbred mouse strain as compared to human peripheral blood lymphocytes: a cytogenetic study.

Int J Radiat Biol 1992;62(2):177—186.

10. Yonezawa M, Takeda A, Misonoh J. Acquired radioresistance after low dose X-irradiation in mice. J Radiat Res 1990;31:256—262.

11. Schmid W. The micronucleus test. Mutat Res 1975;31:9—15.

12. Rigaud O, Moustacchi E. Radioadaptation for gene mutation and possible molecular mechanisms of the adaptive response. Mutat Res 1996;358:127—134.

13. Boothman DA, Meyers M, Fukunaga N, Lee SW. Isolation of X-ray inducible transcripts from radioresistant human melanoma cells. Proc Natl Acad Sci USA 1993;90:7200—7204.

14. Belyaev IY, Alipov YD, Yedneral DI. High sensitivity of chromatin conformation state of human leukocytes to low-dose X-rays. Radiat Environ Biophys 1993;32:99—107.

15. Zaichkina SI, Klokov DYu, Rozanova OM, Aptikaeva GF, Akhmadieva AKh, Smirnova EN, Balakin VE. Cytogenetic damage to bone marrow polychromatic erythrocytes of mice exposed in vivo to low-dose gamma-radiation. Russ J Genet 1998;34(7):1113—1116.

Radioadaptive survival response in mice

Morio Yonezawa

Division of Radiation Biology, Research Institute for Advanced Science and Technology, Osaka Prefecture University, Osaka, Japan

Abstract. Studies (carried out by the author and his collaborators) on the radioadaptive response in mouse survival are reviewed. A priming exposure to an acute dose of X-rays with 0.05−0.10 Gy or 0.30−0.50 Gy induced radioresistance (decrease in bone marrow death rate) in ICR strain mice 2 months or 2 weeks (respectively) after exposure. The intermediate doses of 0.15−0.20 Gy gave no such effects. Partial-body preirradiation experiments showed that the two types of the radioresistance were induced by different mechanisms. Induction of radioresistance was also observed in mice continuously administered with the two radionuclides (^{137}Cs and ^{90}Sr in drinking tap water). These results conflict with the hypothesis of the biological effects of ionizing radiation in which the radiation hazard increases with accumulated dose.

Keywords: biological defense mechanism, bone marrow death, low dose effects, mouse survival, radioadaptive response.

Introduction

Hematopoietic injury has been recognized as an important index of exposure to both mid- and sublethal ionizing radiation and the recovery from radiation injury has been extensively studied. However, little is known about the overshooting recovery in survival rate after multiple exposures in irradiated animals. Maisin et al. [1] first reported that preirradiation of young rats (with as low as 5 R of X-rays) increased the 30-day survival rate when the animals were again exposed to a midlethal dose about 2.5 months later. Though the increment was not significant, the study suggested the possibility of a modifying effect (of low-dose exposure) on the radiosensitivity of whole animals. On the other hand, there are several reports on the induction of radioresistance in mice preirradiated with much higher doses. Daquisto [2] and Nuzhdin et al. [3] noted that a priming dose of 50−150 R induced radioresistance when the mice were again irradiated with midlethal X-rays about 2 weeks later. Bets [4] reported a much higher priming dose, up to 500 R. However, in their experiments, early deaths were observed prior to the onset of bone marrow deaths (i.e., prior to 10 days after midlethal irradiation), presumably induced by infection of some *Pseudomonas* bacteria [5]. Daquisto [2] analyzed the spleen and the thymus, but could not obtain any clue as to the mechanism of the acquired radioresistance.

Address for correspondence: Morio Yonezawa, Division of Radiation Biology, Research Institute for Advanced Science and Technology, Osaka Prefecture University, 1-2 Gakuen-cho, Sakai, Osaka 599-8750, Japan. Tel.: +81-722-54-9855. Fax: +81-722-54-9855. E-mail: yonezawa@riast.osakafu-u.ac.jp

The experiment was carried out to confirm the acquired radioresistance using *Pseudomonas*-free mice (presuming that the clean animals would give reproducible results and certain information on the mechanism).

Mice acquired radioresistance 2 months after exposure to 0.05–0.10 Gy of X-rays

ICR strain mice (free from contamination of *Pseudomonas* bacteria) were purchased and kept in a clean conventional environment. They were preirradiated with 0.05 or 0.10 Gy at 6 weeks of age, and again irradiated with a midlethal dose after a 2 month interval. The 30-day survival rate was significantly increased by the preirradiation, indicating that the animals acquired radioresistance. The result was reproducible. A priming dose of 0.025 Gy proved insufficient, and that of 0.15 Gy overdose [6]. The radioresistance was not observed when the mice were again exposed to a midlethal dose 1 day, 2 weeks, 3 weeks, 1 month, or 1.5 months after the preirradiation with 0.05 Gy. The resistence continued for half a month, 2–2.5 months, but diminished 3 months later, and did not reappear 4 or 5 months later [7].

Induction of radioresistance by preirradiation with 0.3–0.5 Gy

Another type of acquired radioresistance was tested: radioresistance which was induced after a 2-week interval by preirradiation with a much higher dose (as reported by Daquisto [2] and Nuzhdin et al. [3]). Mice were preirradiated with 0.5 Gy of X-rays, and again irradiated with a midlethal dose 2 weeks later. The 30-day survival rate was significantly increased by the preirradiation. A preirradiation dose of 0.3 Gy (which has not yet been reported for acquired radioresistance) also gave a positive result. The radioresistance was not observed in the case of 4- or 5-week and 2-month intervals [7].

Radioresistance was not induced after exposure to 0.15–0.2 Gy

To examine the effect of preirradiation at an intermediate dose, a priming dose of 0.2 Gy was applied. Mice were again irradiated at intervals of 2–5 weeks. The priming dose of 0.2 Gy did not induce any radioresistance 2, 3, 4, or 5 weeks later [7]. As noted previously, a priming exposure to 0.15 Gy 2 months prior to the challenging irradiation gave no radioresistance [6]. The presence of an inert intermediate-dose window indicates that the mechanism for the induction of radioresistance (with the priming dose of 0.05–0.1 Gy) should be different from that with the priming dose of 0.3–0.5 Gy. The dose-effect relation, as illustrated in Fig. 1, shows that the biological effects of ionizing radiation may be distinguished within the following (four) radiation dose ranges: below 0.025 Gy (no acquired radioresistance 2 months later), 0.05–0.10 Gy (significant radioresistance 2–2.5 months later), 0.15–0.20 Gy (no acquired radioresistance

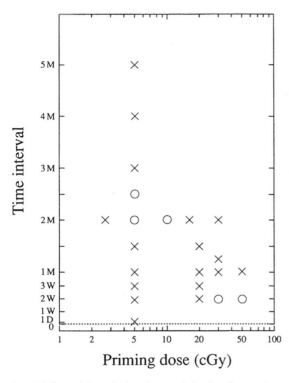

Fig. 1. Effect of the priming dose and the time interval on the acquired radioresistance in mice of ICR strain. ○, significant radioresistance (p < 0.05); ×, insignificant (p > 0.05).

2 weeks to 2 months later), and 0.30–0.50 Gy (significant radioresistance 2 weeks later).

Effect of partial preirradiation on acquired radioresistance

Low-dose effects were reported by Miyachi et al. [8] on the reduction of aggressive behavior in relation to brain serotonin turnover in mice. They also reported an immediate arousal response of mice to low-dose X-rays and its disappearance by olfactory bulbectomy [9]. The effective dose range was 0.05–0.15 Gy, and a higher dose (above 0.25 Gy) induced no such effects. The two reports suggested the testing of partial-body preirradiation to us. Fig. 2 shows the survival rates after the second exposure to a midlethal dose of 8.0 Gy 2 months after partial-body preirradiation with 0.05 Gy. The survival rates on day 30 after the second exposure of the sham-irradiated control group, the whole-body preirradiated group, the head and trunk preirradiated groups, were 30.0 (15/50), 71.9 (41/57), 46.0 (23/50) and 49.0% (24/49), respectively. Only the whole-body preirradiated group showed a significant (p < 0.001, χ^2 test applying Yates' correction) increase in the survival rate. Preirradiation of the head or the trunk was

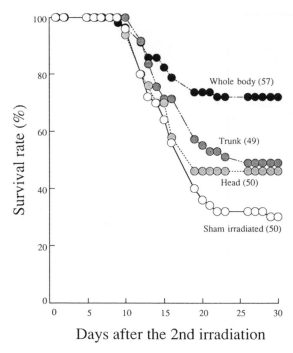

Fig. 2. Survival rates of ICR mice partially irradiated with the priming dose of 0.05 Gy of X-rays 2 months prior to the challenging irradiation. Numbers in parenthesis represent the number of mice used.

not sufficient to induce radioresistance. On the other hand (in case of preirradiation with 0.50 Gy) the 30-day survival rates after the second irradiation with 7.35 Gy of the trunk preirradiated group, head preirradiated group, whole-body, and sham-irradiated group were 67.5 (27/40), 57.5 (23/40), 42.5 (17/40), and 32.0% (16/50), respectively (Fig. 3). Mice acquired the radioresistance by an exposure to the trunk (p < 0.01) more effectively than to the whole body. The result was reproducible (data not shown). The reason why preirradiation of the trunk had a greater effect than that of whole-body preirradiation remains to be clarified. The two types of acquired radioresistance are also distinguished by the partial-body exposure experiments.

The mice seem to receive the four dose ranges of X-rays (mentioned above) as different biological stimuli.

Acquired radioresistance by continuous irradiation from internal radionuclides

Considering the health effects of environmental radiation, many will agree as to the importance of studying whether a radioadaptive response is induced by chronic radiation in whole animals. There is an old report [10] on radioresistance in mice induced by continuous administration with ^{137}Cs and ^{90}Sr in drinking

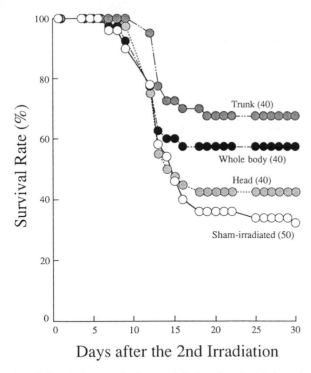

Fig. 3. Survival rates of mice partially irradiated with the priming dose of 0.50 Gy of X-rays 2 weeks prior to the second irradiation with 7.35 Gy. Numbers in parenthesis represent the number of mice used.

tap water after their birth (through their mothers). Mice of NA-2 strain were divided into four groups. Group I, fed with 0.4 µCi/ml of ^{137}Cs and 0.1 µCi/ml of ^{90}Sr, showed reproductive injury, and was not used for the X-irradiation experiment. Groups II and III were administered with 1/10 and 1/100 concentrations of those of group I, respectively. Mice fed with tap water served as the control. The mice were X-irradiated at 7–11 weeks of age. Figure 4 shows the survival rates of male mice after exposure to 600 R of X-rays. Since we could not obtain *Pseudomonas*-free animals during the 1960s, there were early (before day 10 after irradiation) deaths in irradiated animals, presumably caused by the bacterial infection [5]. The 30-day survival rate was improved by the administration of the two radionuclides, markedly in the group III. Similar results were obtained in mice fed with the nuclides through generations (data not shown). Moderate radioresistance in group III was also observed in female mice (data not shown). The results suggest that there might be radioadaptive survival response in mice even after chronic irradiation. Further experimentation, on the effect of external and internal chronic radiation by using *Pseudomonas*-free animals, would be desirable.

98

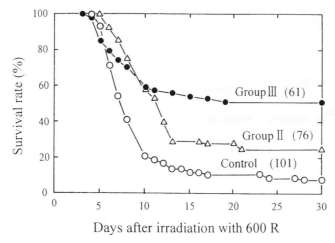

Days after irradiation with 600 R

Fig. 4. Effect of continuous irradiation with internal radionuclides on survival rates of mice after exposure to 600 R of X-rays. Group II was administered from their birth with 0.04 μCi/ml of ^{137}Cs and 0.01 μCi/ml of ^{90}Sr in drinking water. Group III was administered with 1/10 concentrations of those of Group II. The male mice were X-irradiated at 7—10 weeks of age. Numbers in parenthesis represent the number of mice used. (Modified from [10].)

Discussion

Though the radioadaptive response has been extensively studied at the cellular level [11—13], there had been no confirming data (before our reports) that pre-exposure of animals to certain conditioning doses, before exposure with higher challenging doses, decreases bone marrow death rates. The dose-effect relation shows that the biological effects of ionizing radiation to whole animals may be distinguished within the following (four) acute radiation dose ranges: below 0.025 Gy (no acquired radioresistance 2 months later), 0.05—0.10 Gy (significant radioresistance 2—2.5 months later), 0.15—0.20 Gy (no acquired radioresistance 2 weeks to 2 months later), and 0.30—0.50 Gy (significant radioresistance 2 weeks later). Radioresistance has also been induced by internal radiation from the radionuclides (gamma emitter ^{137}Cs and beta emitter ^{90}Sr). Study of the mechanisms of the radioadaptive survival response would lead us to better understand the biological defense mechanisms.

References

1. Maisin J, Van Duyse E, Dunjic A, Van der Merckt J, Wambersie A, Werbrouck D. Acquired radioresistance, radioselection and radioadaptation. In: Buzzati-Traverso AA (ed) Immediate and Low-Level Effects of Ionizing Radiations. London: Taylor & Francis, 1960;183—194.
2. Dacquisto MP. Acquired radioresistance. A review of the literature and report of a confirmatory

experiment. Radiat Res 1959;10:118—129.

3. Nuzhdin NI, Pomeranzeba MD, Kuznezoba NN. Increased resistance of animals to action of ionizing radiation as a result of previous X-ray irradiation. Dokl Akad Nauk SSSR 1960;130: 1359—1361.

4. Betz H. The importance of resistance phase of the organism at the time of application of a lethal dose of X-irradiation. Compt Rend Soc Biol 1950;144: 1439—1442.

5. Flynn RJ. *Pseudomonas aeruginosa* infection and radiobiological research at Argonne national laboratory: effects, diagnosis, epizootiology, control. Laboratory Animal Care 1963;13(1, Part 2):25—35.

6. Yonezawa M, Takeda A, Misonoh J. Acquired radioresistance after low-dose X-irradiation in mice. J Radiat Res 1990;31:256—262.

7. Yonezawa M, Misonoh J, Hosokawa Y. Two types of X-ray induced radioresistance in mice: presence of four dose ranges with distinct biological effects. Mutat Res 1996;358:237—243.

8. Miyachi Y, Kasai H, Ohyama H, Yamada T. Changes of aggressive behavior and brain serotonin turnover after very low dose X-irradiation in mice. Neuro Sci Lett 1994;175:92—94.

9. Miyachi Y, Koizumi T, Yamada T. Immediate arousal response and adaptation to low dose X-rays in mouse and its disappearance by olfactory bulbectomy and nitric oxide inhibitor. Neuro Sci Lett 1994;177:32—34.

10. Megumi T, Yonezawa M, Nishio K. Changes of resistance against X-rays induced by continuous administration of ^{137}Cs and ^{90}Sr in mice. Ann Rep Radiat Ctr Osaka Pref 1968;9:94—97.

11. Olivieri GJ, Bodycote J, Wolff S. Adaptive response of human lymphocytes to low concentrations of radioactive thymidine. Science 1984;223:594—597.

12. Feinendegen LE, Muehlensiepen H, Bond VP, Sondhaus CA. Intracellular stimulation of biochemical control mechanisms by low-LET irradiation. Health Phys 1987;52:663—669.

13. Ikushima T. Chromosomal responses to ionizing radiation reminiscent of an adaptive response in cultured Chinese hamster cells. Mutat Res 1987;180:215—221.

14. Salone B, Pretazzoli V, Bosi A, Olivieri G. Interaction of low-dose irradiation with subsequent mutagenic treatment: role of mitotic delay. Mutat Res 1996;358:155—160.

15. Wolff S. Aspects of the adaptive response to very low doses of radiation and other agents. Mutat Res 1996;358:135—142.

Suppression of ROS-related disease in mouse models by low-dose γ-ray irradiation

Takaharu Nomura[1], Kazuo Sakai[1], Shuji Kojima[2], Mareyuki Takahashi[3] and Kiyonori Yamaoka[4]

[1] *Bio-Science Department Komae Branch, Abiko Research Laboratory, Central Research Institute of Electric Power Industry, Tokyo;* [2] *Research Center for Advanced Science and Technology, University of Tokyo, Tokyo;* [3] *Research Institute for Biosciences, Science University of Tokyo, Chiba; and* [4] *Faculty of Health Sciences, Okayama University Medical School, Okayama, Japan*

Abstract. We examined the effect of low-dose (50 cGy) irradiation on some reactive oxygen species (ROS) related diseases such as fatty liver, Parkinson's disease, and insulin-dependent diabetes mellitus (IDDM) in mouse models. Models for fatty liver and Parkinson's disease were made by injection of chemical agents. Nonobese diabetic (NOD) mice were used as IDDM models.

The low-dose irradiation decreased the level of lipid peroxide in the liver of the fatty-liver model animals. The liver glutathione content was higher in the irradiated group than in the sham-irradiated group. The activity of transaminases (glutamic oxaloacetic transaminase and glutamic pyruvic transaminase), which had been increased by the induction of fatty liver, returned to normal levels more rapidly in the irradiated group than in the sham-irradiated group. Similar effects were observed in the brain of the Parkinson's disease model. The onset of diabetes was later (and the incidence lower) in irradiated NOD mice than in control mice.

These results indicate that ROS-related diseases were suppressed (or inhibited) by 50 cGy of γ-rays and would imply that the low-dose irradiation might be effective in clinical prevention and/or treatment of this kind of disease.

Keywords: endogenous antioxidant materials, fatty liver, insulin-dependent diabetes mellitus, low-dose ionizing radiation, Parkinson's disease.

Background

It is well known that cells have evolved effective defense systems, enzymatic and nonenzymatic mechanisms, against reactive oxygen species (ROS) [1—6]. Glutathione (GSH) is one of the endogenous nonenzymatic antioxidant molecules. GSH levels are reduced in patients with ROS-related diseases. Lowered GSH contents have generally been considered as an index of increased ROS formation, and the GSH depletion in mammalian cells would cause cell damage.

It has generally been considered that any dose of irradiation, however low, should be detrimental to living organisms. Recently, however, it has been shown

Address for correspondence: Dr Takaharu Nomura, Bio-Science Department Komae Branch, Abiko Research Laboratory, Central Research Institute of Electric Power Industry, 2-11-1 Iwado-kita, Komae, Tokyo 201-8511, Japan. Tel.: +81-3-3480-2111. Fax: +81-3-3480-3539.
E-mail: nomura@criepi.denken.or.jp

that low-dose irradiation (under 1 Gy) could induce various stimulating outcomes such as increases in resistance to oxygen toxicity [7], and enhancement of immune functions [8]. We previously reported that 50 cGy of γ-rays increased the level of antioxidant substances (such as superoxide dismutase, catalase, and GSH) in various organs of normal mice, and lowered lipid peroxide levels [1−4]. These findings suggested the possibility that ROS-related disease might be inhibited or suppressed by low-dose irradiation.

To examine this hypothesis, we investigated the effects of low-dose γ-ray irradiation on ROS-related diseases, such as fatty liver, Parkinson's disease, and insulin-dependent diabetes mellitus (IDDM) in mouse models of these diseases.

Materials and Methods

Disease model animals

The C57BL/6 mouse (female, 8 weeks of age) was used as the model for fatty liver and Parkinson's disease. Fatty liver was induced by intraperitoneal administration of carbon tetrachloride (CCl_4) (4 ml/kg of 5% solution in olive oil). Transient hepatocellular disorder is induced by trichloromethyl radicals [9]. Parkinson's-like disease was induced by subcutaneous injection of 1-methyl-4-phenyl-1,2,3,6-tetrahydrpyridine (MPTP) (30 mg/kg) [10]. The toxicity of MPTP is attributed to ROS induced by metabolized MPTP.

For the study on IDDM, we used female nonobese diabetic (NOD) mice. This mouse develops type I diabetes at 14−15 weeks of age, and the incidence of diabetes reaches 80% at 25 weeks of age. IDDM is characterized by the progressive loss of insulin producing pancreatic β-cells by autoimmune mechanisms [11].

The experiments were done following the Guidelines for the Care and Use of Laboratory Animals established by Ministry of Education, Science, Sport and Culture, Japan.

Irradiation

Whole-body irradiation of mice was carried out using 50 cGy of γ-rays from a ^{137}Cs source. The dose rate was 1.17 Gy/min.

Biochemical assays

The activities of glutamic oxaloacetic transaminase (GOT), and glutamic pyruvic transaminase (GPT) in plasma were analyzed (as described previously [9]). Lipid peroxidation levels and total GSH (oxidized and reduced forms) content in the (whole) tissue were also examined [9,10]. Appearance of urine glucose was monitored every week using urine test strips.

Results

Fatty liver

The fatty-liver model mouse was irradiated 24 h after the CCl₄ injection. The histopathological observation is shown in Fig. 1. The livers of the sham-irradiated mice were yellowish, showing fatty degeneration (Fig. 1A). On the other hand, the livers of the irradiated mice were red and looked almost recovered (Fig. 1B).

As shown in Fig. 1, plasma transaminase (GOT and GPT) activities in the irradiated group returned to normal values more rapidly than those of the sham-irradiated group.

Lipid peroxide levels in the liver decreased remarkably after the irradiation (Fig. 2A). On the other hand, the total GSH content of the irradiated group increased more rapidly than that of the sham-irradiated group (Fig. 2B).

Parkinson's disease

The (low-dose) irradiation was carried out 1 h before the administration of MPTP. The lipid peroxide level in the (whole) brain increased remarkably post-

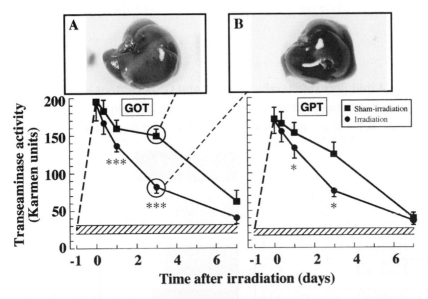

Fig. 1. Effects of γ-ray irradiation (50 cGy) on livers of CCl₄-induced mice. Changes in the glutamic oxaloacetic transaminase (GOT) and the glutamic pyruvic transaminase (GPT) activities of serum of CCl₄-induced mouse after γ-ray irradiation. The area marked with diagonal lines indicates the mean ± SE of the normal group. Each value is the mean ± SE for 4–6 mice. Significantly different from the value of sham-irradiation group at p < 0.05 (*) and p < 0.005 (***). Inserted photographs show the recovery of fatty liver degeneration 3 days after irradiation. **A:** CCl₄ administration only (sham-irradiation mouse). **B:** CCl₄ administration and irradiation (irradiation mouse).

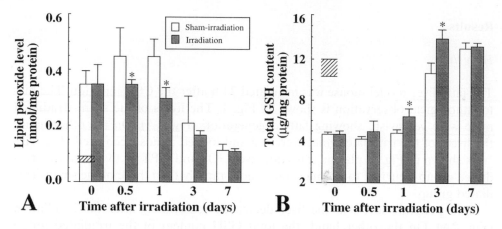

Fig. 2. Effects of γ-ray irradiation on lipid peroxide level (**A**) and total glutathione (oxidized and reduced form) content (**B**) in CCl₄-induced mouse liver. The area marked with diagonal lines indicates the mean ± SE of the normal group. Significantly different from the value of the sham-irradiation group at $p < 0.05$ (*).

treatment with MPTP (Fig. 3A). The increase was significantly suppressed by the γ-ray irradiation. As shown in Fig. 3B, MPTP treatment significantly reduced the total GSH content, while the γ-ray irradiation increased the content.

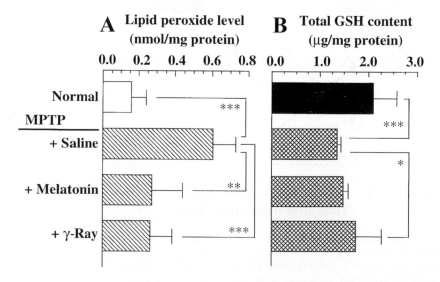

Fig. 3. Effects of γ-ray irradiation on lipid peroxide level (**A**) and total glutathione (oxidized and reduced form) content (**B**) in MPTP-induced mouse brain. Significantly different from the value of the sham-irradiation group at $p < 0.05$ (*), $p < 0.01$ (**) and $p < 0.005$ (***).

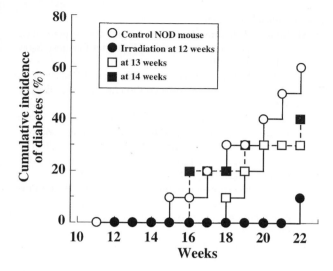

Fig. 4. Effect of a single dose of γ-ray irradiation on incidence of diabetes in NOD mouse. Each value is 10 mice.

Insulin-dependent diabetes mellitus (IDDM)

The NOD mice were irradiated at 12, 13, or 14 weeks of age with 50 cGy γ-rays. The irradiation at 12 weeks of age obviously suppressed the onset of IDDM (Fig. 4). Incidence of diabetes in the NOD mice is caused by the apoptotic death of pancreatic β-cells [12]; the apoptotic cell death, in turn, was caused by the induction of superoxide. We have preliminary data that the low-dose irradiation increased the superoxide peroxidase level in the pancreas of NOD mice. Therefore, the low-dose irradiation might, by increasing antioxidant defense, reduce the superoxide level and suppress the onset of IDDM.

Conclusion

Irradiation with 50 cGy of γ-rays increased the level of endogenous antioxidant materials and suppressed the tissue damage in ROS-related disease (mouse) models. The low-dose irradiation might be effective for prevention and/or treatment of ROS-related diseases.

References

1. Yamaoka K, Edamatsu R, Mori A. Increased SOD activities and decreased lipid peroxide levels induced by low dose X-irradiation in rat organs. Free Radic Biol Med 1991;11:299–306.
2. Yamaoka K, Komoto Y, Suzuka I, Edamatsu R, Mori A. Effect of radon inhibition on biological function - lipid peroxide level, superoxide dismutase activity and membrane fluidity. Arch Biochem Biophys 1993;302:37–41.
3. Matsuki O, Nomura T, Kojima S, Kubodera A. Effect of small-dose γ-ray on endogenous antiox-

idant enzymes in mice. Radioisotopes 1998;47:291—299.

4. Yamaoka K, Kojima S, Takahashi M, Nomura T, Iriyama K. Change of glutathione peroxidase synthesis along with that of superoxide dismutase synthesis in mice spleen after low-dose X-ray irradiation. Biochim Biophys Acta 1998;1381:265—270.

5. Kojima S, Matsuki O, Nomura T, Kubodera A, Honda Y, Honda S, Tanooka H, Wakasugi H, Yamaoka K. Induction of mRNAs for glutathione synthesis-related proteins in mouse liver by low doses of γ-rays. Biochim Biophys Acta 1998;1381:312—318.

6. Kojima S, Matsuki O, Nomura T, Shimura N, Kubodera A, Yamaoka K, Tanooka H, Wakasugi H, Honda Y, Honda S, Sasaki T. Localization of glutathione and induction of glutathione synthesis-related proteins in mouse brain by low doses of γ-rays. Brain Res 1998;808:262—269.

7. Lee YJ, Ducoff HS. Radiation-enhanced resistance to oxygen: a possible relationship to radiation-enhanced longevity. Mech Aging Devel 1984;27:101—109.

8. Liu SZ, Liu WH, Sun JB. Radiation hormesis: its expression in the immune system. Health Phys 1987;52:579—583.

9. Nomura T, Yamaoka K. Low-dose γ-ray irradiation reduces oxidative damage induced by CCl_4 in mouse liver. Free Radic Biol Med 1999;(In press).

10. Kojima S, Matsuki O, Nomura T, Yamaoka K, Takahashi M, Niki E. Elevation of antioxidant potency in the brain of mice by low-dose of γ-ray irradiation and its effect on 1-methyl-4-phenyl-1,2,3,6-tetrahydropyridine (MPTP)-induced brain damage. Free Radic Biol Med 1999;26:388—395.

11. Yoon J-W, Jun H-S, Santamaria P. Cellular and molecular mechanisms for the initiation and progression of β-cell destruction resulting from the collaboration between macrophages and T cells. Autoimmunity 1998;27:109—122.

12. O'Brien BA, Harmon BV, Cameron DP, Allan DJ. Apoptosis is the mode of β-cell death responsible for the development of IDDM in the nonobese diabetic mouse. Diabetes 1997;46:750—757.

Activation of macrophages by low-dose in vivo γ-irradiation and its mechanism

Rensuke Goto and Yuko Ibuki

Laboratory of Radiation Biology, Graduate School of Nutritional and Environmental Sciences, University of Shizuoka, Japan

Abstract. The concanavalin A-induced proliferation of splenocyte obtained from mice after γ-irradiation was enhanced at 2 cGy, but was inhibited at 20 cGy. This enhanced proliferation was found to be caused by the activation of macrophages, but not by the activation of spleno-lymphocytes. The low-dose irradiated macrophages produced more nitric oxide, and showed cytolytic activity against tumor cells. This activation could not be found after in vitro irradiation.

Since we expected that macrophages were activated due to the recognition of oxidized substances formed by in vivo irradiation, we tried to coculture them with irradiated erythrocyte ghosts. No alteration could be found in the accessory function of macrophages. Furthermore, the mRNA expression of cytokines released from macrophages and lymphocytes was determined by RT-PCR. The enhancement of expression of interleukin-1β mRNA in macrophages was induced by both in vivo and in vitro low-dose irradiation, whereas interferon-γ mRNA in spleno-lymphocytes was found only in in vivo irradiation.

Based on these observations, we propose that the in vivo activation of macrophages was caused by the paracrine induction of some cytokines (being initiated with interleukin-1β released slightly from the irradiated macrophages) and by interaction with neighboring cells such as lymphocytes.

Keywords: interferon-γ, interleukin-1, nitric oxide, paracrine, proliferation.

Introduction

Low-doses of ionizing radiation have been known to enhance immune functions. It was reported that chronic low-dose whole body irradiation augmented the splenic proliferative response, and the target cells were T cells [1]. Plaque-forming cell reaction of the spleen was found to be stimulated by single and continuous exposure of X-rays in vivo [2]. Mitogen-induced proliferation of rat splenocyte was also stimulated by in vivo irradiation [3]. However, the mechanism of enhancement has not been investigated sufficiently.

Splenocyte consists of spleno-lymphocytes and accessory cells including macrophages (Mφ) and dendritic cells. Macrophages have not been considered to be target cells by low-dose irradiation because of their radioresistance, but play an important role in the immune responses. Therefore, the effects of low-dose in vivo irradiation on Mφ were investigated.

Address for correspondence: Rensuke Goto, Laboratory of Radiation Biology, Graduate School of Nutritional and Environmental Sciences, University of Shizuoka, 52—1, Yada, Shizuoka-shi 422—8526, Japan. Tel.: +81-54-264-5799. Fax: +81-54-264-5799. E-mail: gotor@sea.u-shizuoka-ken.ac.jp

We examined the mitogen-induced proliferation of splenocyte obtained from mice after low-dose γ-irradiation and found that Mφ were activated by the exposure. Furthermore, this paper describes the alteration of functions and the mechanism of activation of Mφ by low-dose in vivo irradiation.

Materials and Methods

γ-irradiation

Mice (C57BL/6, 7 weeks of age) were irradiated with various doses of γ-rays in an Irradiation Exposure System (Pony Atomic Industry, PS-600SR, 137Cs:22.2TBq). Whole-body irradiation below 4 cGy was given at a dose rate of 0.2 cGy/min, and above 4 cGy at 20 cGy/min.

Preparation of splenocyte, spleno-lymphocytes, and peritoneal Mφ

These cells were prepared according to the procedure as described in a previous paper [4].

Concanavalin A-induced proliferation of splenocyte, and a mixture of spleno-lymphocytes and Mφ

Splenocyte (100 μl, 5×10^6 cells/ml) was placed in the wells of 96-well flat-bottom plates and incubated for 48 h at 37°C in a humidified incubator with 5% CO_2, in the presence of concanavalin A (Con A, 2 μg/ml). ^{3}H-thymidine (370 kBq/ml, 555 GBq/mmol) was added at 9.25 kBq/well 4 h before the termination of culture. Cells were collected and the radioactivity was determined with a liquid scintillation counter (Aloka LSC-3100).

A mixture of spleno-lymphocytes (100 μl, 5×10^6 cells/ml) and peritoneal Mφ (50 μl, 1×10^5 cells/ml) was cultured at 37°C for 48 h in the presence of Con A (50 μl, 8 μg/ml). ^{3}H-thymidine was added 15 h before cell harvest, and the mixture was treated as described above.

Measurement of nitric oxide produced from Mφ

NO_2 concentration was determined using Griess reagent as a portion of nitric oxide (NO) produced [5].

Cytolytic activity of Mφ against tumor cells

Cytolytic activity was determined according to the method described by Higuchi et al. [6]. Briefly, the unirradiated or irradiated Mφ (5×10^4 cells/well) were activated with interferon-γIFN-γ/lipopolysaccharide(LPS) in the wells of 96-well flat-bottom plates for 24 h. Then ^{3}H-thymidine-labeled P815 mastocytoma cells (200 µl, 1×10^5 cells/well) were added to each well. After 24 h, the radioactivity released in supernatant from target cells was determined with a liquid scintillation counter.

Preparation of oxidized or irradiated erythrocyte-ghosts and their effect on the accessory function of Mφ

Erythrocytes were lysed in 30 volumes of a hypotonic hemolysis buffer (10 mM Tris-HCl, pH 7.4). Then they were treated with 5 mM t-butyl hydroperoxide (BHP) for 30 min or with 4 and 400 cGy irradiation in RPMI1640 medium at 37°C and cocultured with Mφ for 1 h at 37°C. The accessory function of treated Mφ for the proliferation of spleno-lymphocytes was measured as described above.

Determination of IL-1β mRNA in Mφ and IFN-γ mRNA in spleno-lymphocytes by RT-PCR

In an in vivo radiation experiment, spleno-lymphocytes and Mφ were prepared 4 h after whole-body irradiation. On the other hand, in an in vitro irradiation, they were allowed to stand in a 5% CO_2 incubator at 37°C for 24 h after preparation, then irradiated and kept in a CO_2 incubator for 1h.

Poly (A)$^+$ mRNA was isolated using QuickPrep Micro mRNA purification kit (Pharmacia Biotec, USA). RT-PCR was performed using the GeneAmp RNA-PCR reaction kit (Perkin Elmer, USA) following the manufacturer's recommended procedures. The cycles of denaturation (95°C, 15 s), annealing (59°C, 30 s), and extension (72°C, 15 s) were continued for 25−30 rounds. Samples were electrophoresed in 2.5% agarose gel containing 0.1 mg/ml of ethidium bromide and visualized with a UV illuminator.

Statistics

The experiments were repeated two or three times. Values are the means of measurements (n = 4∼15). Student's t test was used to determine the significance between the groups.

Results and Discussion

Effects of low-dose in vivo irradiation on proliferation of splenocyte [4]

Figure 1 shows the Con A-induced proliferation of splenocyte obtained from C57BL/6 mice after γ-irradiation. The irradiation of 2 cGy significantly enhanced the proliferation of splenocyte, though 20 cGy irradiation lowered its response. This enhancement agrees with the reports by Liu et al. [2] and Ishii et al. [3].

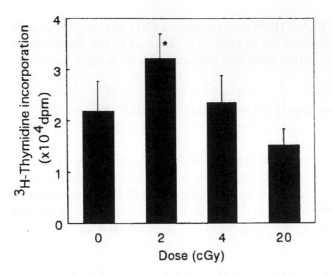

Fig. 1. Dose response in proliferation of splenocytes obtained from γ-irradiated mice; * = $p < 0.05$.

As stated earlier, splenocyte consists of spleno-lymphocytes and accessory cells including Mφ and dendritic cells. Accessory cells play an important role in the spleno-lymphocyte response to Con A [7]. We noted Mφ as accessory cells, and investigated as to which was more affected by low-dose irradiation, spleno-lymphocytes or Mφ. First, we examined the proliferation of irradiated spleno-lymphocytes cultured with unirradiated peritoneal Mφ in the presence of Con A. The spleno-lymphocytes were prepared 4 h after in vivo irradiation. The peritoneal Mφ were used instead of spleno-Mφ, because it was difficult to isolate the

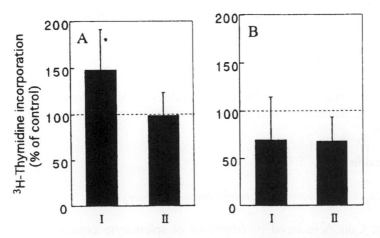

Fig. 2. Proliferation of spleno-lymphocytes obtained from low-dose γ-irradiated mice. **A:** 2 cGy γ-irradiation. **B:** 20 cGy γ-irradiation; I = irradiated splenocytes; II = irradiated spleno-lymphocytes + unirradiated Mφ; * = $p < 0.05$.

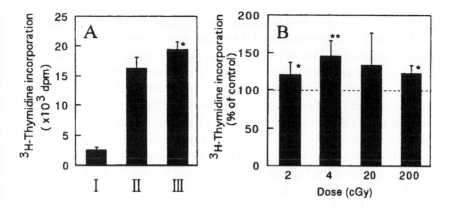

Fig.3. **A:** Effect of irradiated Mφ on proliferation of unirradiated spleno-lymphocytes, I = spleno-lymphocytes; II = spleno-lymphocytes + unirradiated Mφ; III = spleno-lymphocytes + irradiated Mφ (2 cGy); * = p < 0.05 (vs. II). **B:** Dose response of irradiated Mφ, * = p < 0.05; ** = p < 0.01.

dendritic cell-free spleno-Mφ from splenocyte in a short time.

The proliferative response of spleno-lymphocytes irradiated at 2 cGy was almost the same as that of the unirradiated control (Fig. 2A), and different from that of irradiated splenocyte (Fig. 1). In the case of 20 cGy irradiation, both responses decreased (Fig. 2B). These results show that the spleno-lymphocytes were hardly affected by 2 cGy irradiation, but damaged by 20 cGy. Furthermore, the proliferation of unirradiated spleno-lymphocytes was examined in the presence of in vivo irradiated peritoneal Mφ. As shown in Fig. 3A, spleno-lympho-

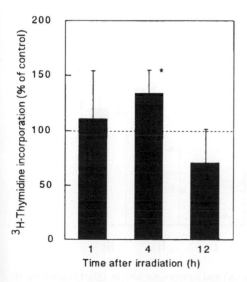

Fig. 4. Effect of Mφ on proliferation of spleno-lymphocytes as a function of time after γ-irradiation, * = p < 0.05.

cytes showed a low level of ^{3}H-thymidine incorporation. The response was increased by the addition of unirradiated Mφ, and more significantly enhanced by the addition of irradiated Mφ. We carried out similar experiments using Mφ prepared from mice that received several doses of irradiation (2 cGy to 200 cGy). The proliferation of spleno-lymphocytes was enhanced especially at 4 cGy, and even at 20 cGy, although 20 cGy irradiation depressed the proliferation of irradiated splenocytes (Fig. 1B). These results suggest that the enhancement of proliferation of spleno-lymphocytes by low-dose irradiation is caused not by the activation of spleno-lymphocytes, but by the activation of spleno-Mφ. The response of the spleno-lymphocytes was the highest in the presence of Mφ prepared 4 h after irradiation, and decreased after 12 h, indicating that a given time is required for the activation of Mφ (Fig. 4).

Functional changes of Mφ by low-dose irradiation

Since the activation of Mφ by low-dose irradiation was observed, we have investigated the functional changes of Mφ. Irradiated Mφ produced more nitric oxide than unirradiated Mφ in the presence of IFN-γ and/or LPS) (Fig. 5A) [8].

Nitric oxide has been known to mediate the cytolytic activity of Mφ against tumor cells by inhibiting DNA synthesis, mitochondorial respiration and the Krebs cycle [9,10]. Therefore, the cytolytic activity of Mφ activated by low-dose irradiation against P-815 mastocytoma cells was investigated (Fig. 5B). Mφ treated with 10 U of INF-γ and LPS increased greatly the cytolytic activity as well as the amounts of NO, and the low-dose irradiation enhanced the cytolytic activity even more.

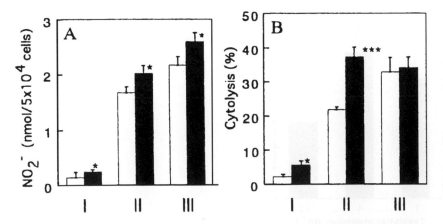

Fig. 5. NO production from low-dose irradiated Mφ **(A)** and its cytolytic activity **(B)**. I = nontreated; II = IFN-γ (10U) + LPS; III = IFN-γ (100U) + LPS; □ = control; ■ = 4 cGy; * = p < 0.05; ** = p < 0.01; *** = p < 0.001.

Effect of low-dose in vitro irradiation on Mφ [4]

To determine whether the observed effects of low-dose in vivo irradiation on Mφ is direct or indirect, we tried in vitro irradiation. No enhancement of proliferation of spleno-lymphocytes was observed in the presence of Mφ irradiated in vitro with various doses of γ-rays (data not shown). Nitric oxide production was not enhanced by low-dose in vitro irradiation (data not shown). These results indicate that the low-dose in vivo irradiation may affect Mφ indirectly.

Ionizing radiation is known to induce oxidative damage in cell membrane such as lipid peroxidation. The erythrocytes modified by oxidizing agents have been reported to cause lipid peroxydation and to be adherent to Mφ [11]. We considered that Mφ might be activated to remove oxidative substances produced by low-dose irradiation and tried to coculture Mφ with irradiated or oxidized erythrocyte ghosts. The accessory function of Mφ treated with oxidized (BHP) or irradiated (4 and 400 cGy) erythrocyte-ghosts did not change (Fig. 6), indicating that the accessory function of Mφ was hardly activated by recognition of oxidized substances.

Release of cytokines from Mφ and spleno-lymphocytes by low-dose irradiation

Ionizing radiation and oxidative injury has been reported to enhance the release of interleukin-1 (IL-1) from Mφ and monocytes [12−15]. IL-1 leads to the B

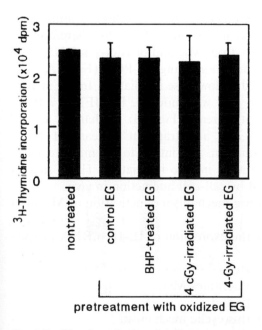

Fig. 6. Proliferation of spleno-lymphocytes cocultured with peritoneal Mφ pretreated with oxidized erythrocytes-ghosts(EG).

114

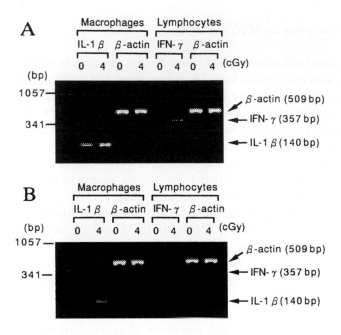

Fig. 7. Expression of IL-1β mRNA in peritoneal Mφ and IFN-γ mRNA in spleno-lymphocytes obtained from low-dose irradiated mice **(A)** and irradiated in vitro **(B)**.

cell proliferation [16,17] and T cell activation [17—19]. In response to some cytokines, lymphocytes produced IFN-γ which activates Mφ [20]. Therefore, we investigated the expression of IL-1mRNA from Mφ and of IFN-γ mRNA from spleno-lymphocytes 4 h after in vivo irradiation using RT-PCR (Fig. 7A). The expression of both mRNAs was increased by low-dose irradiation. In the in vitro irradiation, IL-1β mRNA expression in Mφ was induced, but IFN-γ mRNA expression in spleno-lymphocytes did not increase (Fig. 7B). Ishihara et al. [13] have already reported the immediate, early, and transient increase of IL-1β mRNA in spleen cells after in vitro irradiation, in contrast to the mediate, early, and continuous (not transient) increase after in vivo irradiation. These suggest the regulatory mechanisms are mediated by cell-cell interaction in vivo.

In conclusion, we proposed the following mechanism of activation of Mφ after low-dose in vivo irradiation:

1) low-dose irradiation slightly induces the expression of IL-1β mRNA in spleno-Mφ;
2) the IL-1β stimulates spleno-lymphocytes;
3) the lymphocytes release IFN-γ, which activates Mφ;
4) the activated Mφ produce more IL-1β; and
5) lastly, Mφ are activated gradually by this cyclic mechanism.

Some other lymphokines released from the activated lymphocytes such as interleukin-2 may also participate in the activation of Mφ.

Acknowledgements

This work was supported by the Hayashi Memorial Foundation for Female Natural Scientists and by the Researh Foundation for the Electrotechnology of Chubu.

References

1. James SJ, Makinodan T. T cell potentiation in normal autoimmune-prone mice after extended exposure to low doses of ionizing radiation and/or caloric restriction. Int J Radiat Biol 1988; 53:137—152.
2. Liu SZ, Liu WH, Sun JB. Radiation hormesis: its expression in the immune system. Health Phys 1987;52:579—583.
3. Ishii K, Muto N, Yamamoto I. Augmentation in mitogen-induced proliferation of rat splenocytes by low dose whole-body X-irradiation. Nippon Acta Radiologica 1990;50:64—69.
4. Ibuki Y, Goto R. Enhancement of concanavalin A-induced proliferation of spleno-lymphocytes by low-dose-irradiated macrophages. Radiat Res 1994;35:83—91.
5. Ding AH, Nathan CF, Stuehr DJ. Release of reactive nitrogen intermediates and reactive oxygen intermediates from mouse peritoneal macrophages. J Immunol 1988;141:2407—2412.
6. Higuchi M, Higashi N, Taki H, Osawa T. Cytolytic mechanisms of activated macrophages: tumor necrosis factor and L-arginine-dependent mechanisms act synergistically as the major cytolytic mechanisms of activated macrophages. J Immunol 1990;144:1425—1431.
7. Hirayama Y, Inaba K, Komatubara S, Yoshida K, Kawai J, Naito K, Muramatsu S. Accessory cell functions of dendritic cells and macrophages in the thymic T-cell response to Con A. Immunology 1987;62:393—399.
8. Ibuki Y, Goto R. Augmentation of NO production and cytolytic activity of Mφ obtained from mice irradiated with a low dose of γ-rays. Radiat Res 1995;36:209—220.
9. Stuehr DJ, Nathan CF. Nitric oxide: a macrophage product responsible for cytostasis and respiratory inhibition in tumor target cells. J Exp Med 1989;169:1543—1555.
10. Hibbs JB, Taintor RR, Vavrin Z, Rachlin EM. Nitric oxide: a cytotoxic activated macrophage effecter molecule. Biochem Biophys Res Commun 1988;157:87—94.
11. Beppu M, Ochiai H, Kikugawa K. Macrophage recognition of the erythrocytes modified by oxidizing agents. Biochem Biophys Acta 1987;930:244—253.
12. Ishihara H, Tsuneoka K, Dimchev AB, Shikita M. Induction of the expression of the interleukin-1b gene in mouse spleen by ionizing radiation. Radiat Res 1993;133:321—326.
13. Ishihara H, Tanaka I, Nemoto K, Tsuneoka K, Cheeramakara C, Yoshida K, Ohtsu H. Immediate-early, transient induction of the interleukin-1β gene in mouse spleen macrophages by ionizing radiation. Radiat Res 1995;36:112—124.
14. O'Brien-Landner A, Nelson ME, Kimler BF, Wesselius LJ. Release of interleukin-1 by human alveolar macrophages after in vitro irradiation. Radiat Res 1993;136:37—41.
15. Gougerot-Pocidalo M, Roche Y, Fay M, Perianin A, Bailly S. Oxidative injury amplifies interleukin-1-like activity produced by human monocytes. Int J Immunopharmacol 1989;11:961—969.
16. Howard M, Mizel SB, Lachman L, Ansel J, Johnson B, Paul WE. Role of interleukin-1 in anti-immunoglobulin-induced B cell proliferation. J Exp Med 1983;157:1529—1543.
17. Miossec P, Yu C, Ziff M. Lymphocyte chemotastic activity of human interleukin-1. J Immunol 1984;133:2007—2011.
18. Dinarello CA. Interleukin-1 and interleukin-1 antagonism. Blood 1991;77:1627—1652.
19. Hagiwara H, Huang HS, Arai N, Herzenberg LA, Arai K, Zlothik A. Interleukin 1 modulates messenger RNA levels of lymphokines and of other molecules associated with T cell activation in the T cell lymphoma LBRM33-1A5. J Immunol 1987;138:2514—2519.
20. Blach CM, Catterall JR, Remington JS. In vivo and in vitro activation of alveolar macrophages by recombinant interferon-γ. J Immunol 1987;138:491—495.

Induction of glutathione in mouse brain by low doses of γ-rays

Shuji Kojima[1] and Kiyonori Yamaoka[2]

[1]*Research Institute for Biological Sciences, Science University of Tokyo, Chiba; *[2]*Faculty of Health Sciences, Okayama University Medical School, Okayama, Japan*

Abstract. Induction of the in vivo antioxidant activity (following low doses of γ-ray irradiation) was investigated in C57BL/6 mice. Significant elevations in the activity were observed in several organs (including the liver, pancreas, and brain) soon after postirradiation with 50 cGy of γ-rays. As for the brain, changes in the reduced form of glutathione (GSH) level were examined after radiation. The cerebral GSH level increased soon after irradiation with 50 cGy of γ-rays, reaching a maximum 3 h posttreatment. Cerebral GSH levels remained significantly higher than that of the nonirradiated control until 12 h (posttreatment) and had returned to the control level by 24 h. Finally, the induction of mRNAs proteins (involved in the de novo synthesis and regeneration of GSH in the brain) by subjection to low-dose γ-ray irradiation was investigated. The level of mRNA for γ-glutamylcysteine synthetase (a rate limiting enzyme of the de novo pathway) had significantly increased at 0.5 h, and remained high until 2 h postirradiation. The level transiently lowered to the nonirradiated control level at 3 h and slightly increased again after 6 h postirradiation. The level of mRNA for glutathione reductase, a key enzyme of the regeneration cycle, was increased at 0.5 h and peaked strongly at 2 h. Thereafter, the level declined to (almost) that at time 0, 12 h postirradiation. These results indicate that the increase in endogenous GSH in the brain of the mouse soon after low-dose γ-ray irradiation is a consequence of the induction of GSH synthesis-related proteins, and occurs via both the de novo synthesis and the regeneration pathways.

Keywords: glutathione, low-dose γ-rays, mouse brain, mRNA.

Introduction

Pretreatment with small amounts of oxidant induces resistance to subsequent, and otherwise lethal, doses of oxidant. The adaptive responses involve the induction of various molecules, including superoxide dismutase (SOD), glutathione peroxidase, metallothionein, heat-shock protein, and others [1—5]. Though the precise mechanisms of these responses have not been established, the involvement of radical oxygen species (ROS) is suspected. Meanwhile, most of the damaging effects of ionizing radiation are also mediated by ROS, such as hydroxyl radicals and superoxide anion radicals [6,7]. Thus, similar adaptive responses to small amounts of oxidative stress will also be expected in low-doses of ionizing radiation. The induction of SOD has already been reported with respect to the efficacy of low level ionizing radiation on the in vivo antioxidant activity [8—10]. This phenomenon is understandable, because radiation toxicity to living cells is,

Address for correspondence: Shuji Kojima, Research Institute for Biological Sciences, Science University of Tokyo, 2669 Yamazaki, Noda-shi, Chiba 278-0022, Japan. Tel.: +81-471-23-9755. Fax: +81-471-23-9755. E-mail: kjma@rs.noda.sut.ac.jp

in essence, due to ROS generated by the interaction between water molecules and ionizing radiation, and antioxidant enzymes such as SOD are induced under certain conditions of oxygen stress.

In this study, we have focused our attention on endogenous thiol-related antioxidants, in particular the reduced glutathione (GSH), which is involved in the protection of living cells against radiation, oxidative damage, and certain toxic compounds of endogenous and exogenous origins [11–13]. We investigated the effect of low doses of radiation on the induction of antioxidant activity in various tissues of C57BL/6 mice in order to elucidate the additional stimulating effects of low-dose radiation in connection with alterations of GSH content, the related enzymes, and their gene expressions [14–18]. Parts of the work are presented in this article.

Materials and Methods

Female C57BL/6 mice, 8 weeks of age, were purchased from Tokyo Experimental Animals (Tokyo, Japan). They were housed in standard polycarbonate cages with sterilized wood chip bedding and were acclimated to the animal facility environment for 1 week. Mice were allowed free access to water and sterilized normal diet (CE-2, CLEA Co., Ltd., Tokyo, Japan).

Mice were irradiated with γ-rays from a ^{137}Cs source (GAMMACELL 40, Nordin International, Inc., Canada) at a dose of 50 cGy (1.16 Gy/min). Mice were also exposed to different doses of γ-rays and sacrificed 3 h after irradiation. The dose-dependent effect of radiation was examined by analysis of various organs after sacrificing the mice in each instance.

The antioxidant activity of the cytosol (of the various tissues) was estimated from the reaction with a chemically stable radical, 1,1-diphenyl-2-picrylhydrazyl (DPPH). An appropriate volume of the cytosol was added to an ethanol solution containing 0.1 mM DPPH. The reaction mixture was maintained at room temperature for 20 min, and the absorbance was recorded at 517 nm. A reduction of absorbance was regarded as indicating the scavenging activity of each tissue cytosol fraction. The cytosol fraction was prepared using a (slightly) modified method of that of Xia and colleagues [19].

Total glutathione (GSH + GSSG) content in the brain was measured using a modified spectrophotometric technique [20]. The GSH concentration of each sample was calculated in μg/mg protein. The protein content was measured according to the method of Lowry et al [21].

Each brain was homogenized in chilled 10 mM Tris-HCl buffer (pH 7.4) containing 0.32 M sucrose and 1 mM EDTA using a Teflon-glass Potter homogenizer. The homogenate was centrifuged at 36,000g for 30 min at 4°C and the supernatant was used for enzyme assays. The activity of γ-glutamylcysteine synthetase (γ-GCS), the rate-limiting enzyme for de novo GSH biosynthesis, was measured by means of a coupled enzyme assay that evaluates NADH oxidation [22]. The activity of glutathione reductase (GR) was measured spectrophoto-metrically at 340 nm in terms of NADPH oxidation at 30°C [23]. The activity was expressed as nmol of NADPH oxidized/min/mg protein.

Thioredoxin (TRX) content in the brain was measured by means of an insulin-reducing assay [24]. Insulin-reducing activity (U/L) was calculated as micromoles of NADPH oxidized per minute from the following formula [25];

$$Activity\ (U/L) = \Delta A340 \times 0.12 \times 105/6.2$$

Expression of γ-GCS-, GR- and TRX-mRNAs was analyzed by Northern blotting. Total RNA was isolated (from brain kept in a deepfreeze at –120°C) until use by means of the acid guanidium isothiocyanate-phenol-chloroform extraction methods. The RNA was quantified spectrophoto-metrically at 260 nm (the ratio of A260 nm to A280 nm always exceeded 1.8), and 15 μg aliquots of total RNA were size-fractionated by electrophoresis on a 1.0% agarose gel (Nippon Gene, Toyama, Japan). RNA was then blotted onto nylon membrane from the gel using 0.02 M MOPS buffer (pH 7.0), and immobilized by UV cross-linking. The relative amounts of RNA were judged by hybridization with a mouse glyceralde-hyde-3-phosphate dehydrogenase (GAPDH) probe. Specific cDNA probes were obtained as follows. (A mouse GR cDNA was a kind gift from Prof. Dieter Werner, German Cancer Research Center.) Mouse γ-GCS, TRX, and GAPDH cDNAs were synthesized by RT-PCR (Titan, Boehringer Mannheim, Mannheim) from mouse liver total RNA using oligo DNA primers for γ-GCS (5′-CACATC-TACCACGCAGTCA-3′ and 5′-TTCGCTTTTCTAAATCCTGA-3′), TRX (5′-GCAACAGCCAAAATGGTGA-3′ and 5′-GGCAGTTGGGTATAGACTCT-CC-3′), and GAPDH (5′-TGAAGGTCG-GTGTGAACGGATTTGGC-3′ and 5′-CATGTAGGCCATGAGGCCACCAC-3′). cDNA was amplified (35 cycles, 94°C, 1 min; 55°C, 1 min; 72°C, 1 min) and PCR products were subcloned into the pGEM-T vector (Promega, Madison, WI) for amplification. Hybridization was carried out in a solution consisting of 5 × SSPE (20 × SSPE = 3.6 M NaCl, 200 mM NaH_2PO_4, 20 mM EDTA, pH 7.4), 10 × Denhardt's reagent (0.2% Ficoll, 0.2% polyvinylpyrrolidone, 0.2% BSA), 50% formamide, 1.4% sodium dodecyl sulfate (SDS), and 0.1 mg/ml herring sperm DNA with 32p-labeled probes at 42°C. After hybridization, the membrane was washed with 6 × SSC (20 × SSC = 3 M NaCl, 0.3 M trisodium citrate) and 0.1% SDS at 42°C for 30 min, 1 × SSC and 0.1% SDS at 55°C for 30 min, and 0.1 × SSC and 0.1% SDS at 60°C for 30 min. Quantitation was done with a laser image analyser (Fujix BAS 2500, Fuji Film, Kanagawa). The membrane was also exposed to an X-ray film (Fuji HR-HA30, Fuji Film) with an intensifying screen at –80°C.

The data were analyzed using Student's t test. The criterion of significance was taken as $p < 0.05$.

Results

Changes in tissue antioxidant activity after 50 cGy γ-ray irradiation

Induction of the antioxidant activity of various tissues after treatment with low-dose γ-ray irradiation was examined as a function time after a whole-body γ-ray irradiation at a dose of 50 cGy. As shown in Fig .1, significant increases of the activity were observed in some organs, including the liver, pancreas, and brain, early after postirradiation. The pattern varied slightly among organs, and elevations in the liver and brain were maintained for 24 h.

As concerning the liver and the brain, the dose-response relationship between irradiation and antioxidant activity was examined 3 h after irradiation. The activities of both tissues were increased after exposure to 25 and 50 cGy. However, the antioxidant activity was significantly lower at 200 cGy (data not shown). Thereafter, the dose of γ-rays was fixed at 50 cGy throughout the experiment.

Effect of γ-ray on brain glutathione level

As shown in Fig. 2, the total glutathione level of the brain increased soon after irradiation with 50 cGy of γ-rays and reached a maximum at around 3 h post-eqalignno-treatment. It remained significantly higher than the control level until 12 h and (virtually) returned to the nontreated control level 24 h postirradiation.

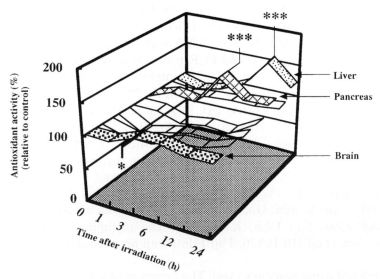

Fig. 1. Changes in the scavenging activity of various tissues after whole body γ-ray irradiation of C57BL/6 mice at a dose of 50 cGy. The activity was assessed by the reaction of the tissue cytosol fractions with DPPH. Each point was indicated as a value relative to that obtained with nonirradiated control tissue cytosol fraction. *, *** Significantly different from the nonirradiated group at $p < 0.05$ and $p < 0.001$, respectively. (Modified from [14].)

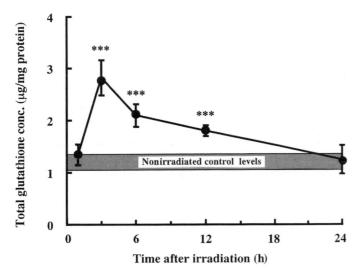

Fig. 2. Total glutathione (GSH + GSSG) levels in the brain of mice after 50 cGy of γ-ray irradiation. Each point indicates the mean ± SD of 5 mice. Each column indicates the mean ± SD of 5 mice. *** Significantly different from each nonirradiated control group at p < 0.001. (Modified from [18].)

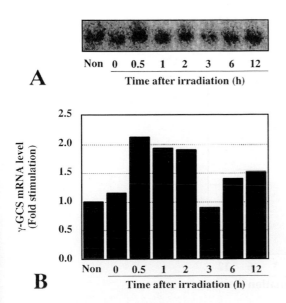

Fig. 3. Changes in γ-GCS mRNA level in the brain of mice after γ-ray irradiation. **A:** Changes in autoradiogram after γ-ray irradiation. **B:** Results of quantification of mRNA levels by densitometric analysis of the upper autoradiogram. Relative mRNA levels are indicated as the ratio of the γ-GCS mRNA level to the mRNA level of the housekeeping gene GAPDH. (Modified from [17].)

Induction of mRNAs for glutathione synthesise-related proteins by γ-rays

GSH is synthesised from its constituent amino acids via two ATP-dependent steps catalysed by γ-GCS and GSH synthetase (GSHS), respectively. GSH is utilized by reaction with free radicals, or in reactions catalysed by glutathione peroxidase (GPX), thereby producing its oxidized form of GSSG. GSH is also regenerated from GSSG in an NADPH-dependent reaction catalysed by GR. Thus, the mRNA levels for proteins involved in the de novo GSH synthesis and regeneration cycle (after irradiation with a low dose of γ-rays) were examined. The expression of the housekeeping gene GAPDH, which served as a control, was approximately the same throughout all of the time courses. First, γ-GCS mRNA was investigated, together with the changes in γ-GCS activity. As shown in Fig. 3, the γ-GCS mRNA level was significantly increased between 0.5 h and 2 h postirradiation. Thereafter, the expression returned to the nonirradiated control level after 3 h, but was again increased 6 and 12 h postirradiation. The γ-GCS activity was increased soon after irradiation, reaching a plateau 3 h postirradiation, and remaining elevated up to 24 h (data not shown).

GR is a key enzyme in the regeneration of GSH from GSSG. As shown in Fig. 4, the induction of GR mRNA was observed at 0.5 h, and reached a maximum

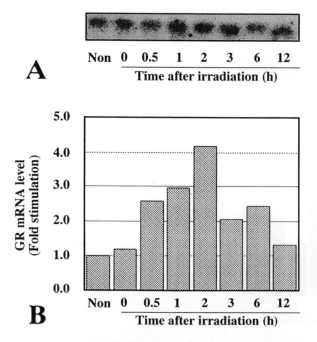

Fig. 4. Changes in GR mRNA level in the brain of mice after γ-ray irradiation. **A:** Changes in autoradiogram after γ-ray irradiation. **B:** Results of quantification of mRNA levels by densitometric analysis of the upper autoradiogram. Relative mRNA levels are indicated as the ratio of the GR mRNA level to the mRNA level of the housekeeping gene GAPDH. (Modified from [17].)

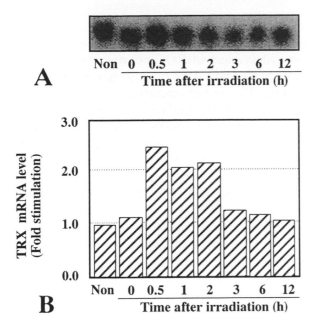

Fig. 5. Changes in TRX mRNA level in the brain of mice after γ-ray irradiation. **A:** Changes in auto-radiogram after γ-ray irradiation. **B:** Results of quantification of mRNA by densitometric analysis of the upper autoradiogram. Relative mRNA levels are indicated as the ratio of the TRX mRNA level to the mRNA level of the housekeeping gene GAPDH. (Modified from [17].)

at 2 h postirradiation. Then, the level gradually declined to almost that of the nonirradiated control 12 h postirradiation. The maximum showed more than a 4-fold degree of stimulation. GR activity was also increased soon after irradiation, reaching a plateau at 3 h, and then remaining high until 24 h (data not shown).

TRX is not only a potential endogenous thiol-containing antioxidant, but also may contributes to the biosynthesis of GSH by promoting cystine transport into cells. As shown in Fig. 5, TRX mRNA level also increased soon after irradiation (50 cGy), peaked at 0.5 h, and then declined almost to the level of the non-irradiated control after 3 h posttreatment. TRX content in the brain of mice was drastically decreased immediately after irradiation, then increased, peaked at 3 h, and quickly declined to near the control level at 6 h postirradiation (data not shown).

Discussion

ROS, such as hydrogen peroxide, hydroxyl radicals, and superoxide anion radicals, are readily generated in many cells by metabolic processes such as respiration, ischemia/reperfusion, and oxidation of fatty acids, and are highly toxic to cells by damaging such components as DNA, lipids, and enzymes. Cells can be injured, and even killed under the most serious of conditions, when the content of ROS exceeds the cellular antioxidant capacity. It is understandable, then, that cells have evolved effective defense systems against ROS, not only through enzymatic mechanisms (such as catalase, SOD, and GPX) but also nonenzymatically via GSH, TRX, and vitamins C and E. The best characterized endogenous antioxidant of these nonenzymatic molecules is GSH. GSH is considered to act as a radical scavenger with the redox-active sulphydryl group reacting with oxidants to produce GSSG, then to be regenerated in a reaction mediated by NADPH and catalyzed by GR [12]. Lowered levels of GSH have generally been considered an index of increased oxidative stress, resulting from the increased formation of ROS and the depletion of GSH from mammalian cells, ultimately causing cell damage due to oxidative stress.

In addition, the induction of antioxidant-related proteins, such as SOD and heat-shock protein (hsp 70), has already been well established in various organisms after treatment with sublethal pressures of oxygen [1—5]. This phenomenon is thought to act as an adaptive stress response, though the complex mechanisms involved have still not been elucidated.

Ionizing radiation can also be considered to be a source of ROS. Therefore, some of the adaptive responses can easily be anticipated after treatment with low-dose radiation. In this study, we first confirmed the induction of the increased antioxidant activity of various tissues after treatment with low-dose γ-ray irradiation. Low doses (25—50 cGy) of γ-ray irradiation significantly increased the scavenging activity of tissues. This phenomenon was seen soon after postirradiation and persisted, suggesting an adaptive response to the ROS generated by the radiation. It was surprising to find that this effect is only seen over a very narrow dose range of radiation and only in certain tissues including the liver, pancreas, and brain. Also, this response varied slightly among the liver, pancreas, and brain, suggesting different sensitivities of these tissues to the radiation. The involvement of enzymatic and nonenzymatic defense systems can be anticipated to contribute to the mechanism of the elevated activity of these organs. In this study, we focused our attention on GSH, which is one of the most abundant and well-characterized endogenous antioxidant. As shown in Fig. 2, the GSH level in the whole brain was significantly elevated by a single 50 cGy dose of γ-rays. However, it is still necessary to examine the alterations of other factors such as vitamins C and E.

Induction of mRNAs for GSH synthesis-related proteins was further examined in order to determine whether the elevation of GSH is a posttranscriptional event. γ-GCS and GR, which are rate-limiting enzymes in the de novo GSH synthesis and the regeneration cycle for GSH synthesis, were induced in (almost) the same fashion by the irradiation. Induction of these mRNAs occurred soon after irradiation (50 cGy), and reached a maximum at between 0.5 and 2 h postirradiation. The activity of both of these enzymes was induced at a later time point than the mRNA expression, and remained high throughout 24 h postirradiation. However, the level of TRX, which contributes to the de novo

GSH biosynthesis by supplying L-cysteine [26], changed differently; the TRX level transiently increased (with a maximum at 3 h) following a significant decrease immediately after irradiation. The time-course of expression of TRX mRNA was similar to those in the cases of proto-oncogenes such as c-fos, c-jun, c-myc, and c-Ha-ras, expression of which is induced at the same dose of γ-rays as in Epstein-Barr virus-transformed human lymphoblastoid 244B cells [27]. Induction of NF-κB after the same dose of γ-rays irradiation has also been demonstrated. This is biologically important, because NF-κB is involved in the induction of many distinct classes of transcription factor. Further, TRX modulates the physiological function of NF-κB in the cytokine expression in various cells [28,29]. TRX has recently been shown to reduce the nuclear factor Ref-1, which in turn increases DNA binding of NF-κB, AP-1, and other transcription factors [30,31]. In view of the significant difference in the elevation of TRX in the brain of mice (in comparison with those of γ-GCS and GR activities) TRX may also have functions other than supplying cysteine for the de novo pathway (as described above). The overall increase of GSH in the brain soon after low-dose γ-ray irradiation is due to operation of both the de novo pathway and the regeneration cycle for GSH synthesis. Contrastingly, in the liver the induction was predominantly via the regeneration cycle and not de novo synthesis [16]. This difference in induction mechanism between brain and liver could be explained by the fact that the content of GSH initially contained in the brain was significantly lower than that in the liver. Therefore, protection of brain tissue from radiation exposure may require a much larger adaptive response than in liver. The induction of transcription after treatment with low doses of ionizing radiation might be part of a complex response by cells to protect themselves against further oxidative injury, or it might be caused by activation of repair mechanisms. It remains to be determined whether different signaling pathways and mechanisms are involved after exposure to different levels of ionizing radiation. Further, each gene response may be linked to a different signaling pathway.

In this study, we have demonstrated that the elevation of GSH content in the brain of mice irradiated with low-doses of γ-rays follows the induction of mRNAs coding for GSH synthesis-related proteins. These results imply that low doses of γ-rays may be useful for clinical prevention and/or therapy of various ROS-related brain disorders such as stroke, Alzheimer's disease, and Parkinson's disease. Preclinical studies of the application of this efficacy towards damages, such as acute hepatopathy and type I diabetes whose pathogenesis is ROS-related, have also been shown by our co-authors.

Acknowledgements

The authors thank Dr Dieter Werner (Institute of Cell and Tumor Biology, German Cancer Research Center, Heiderberg, Federal Republic of Germany) for his kind gift of a glutahione reductase-specific cDNA probe.

This work was supported in part by a Grant-in-Aid for Scientific Research (11680556) from the Ministry of Education, Science, Sports and Culture of Japan.

References

1. Galiazzo F, Schiesser AG, Rotilio G. Glutathione peroxidase in yeast: presence of the enzyme and induction by oxidative conditions. Biochem Biophys Res Commun 1987;147:1200−1205.
2. Jamieson DJ, Rivers SL, Stephen DW. Saccharomyces cerevisiae protein induced by peroxide and superoxide stress. Microbiology 1994;140:3277−3283.
3. Kimball RE, Reddy K, Pierce TH, SchwartzMustafa LW, Cross C. Oxygen toxicity: augmentation of antioxidant defense mechanisms in rat lung. Am J Physiol 1976;230:1425−1431.
4. Shiraishi N, Aono K, Utsumi K. Increased metallothionein content in rat liver induced by X-irradiation and exposure to high oxygen tension. Radiat Res 1983;95:298−302.
5. Williams RS, Thomas JA, Fina M. German Z, Benjamin IJ. Human heat shock protein 70 (hsp 70) protects murine cells from injury during metabolic stress. J Clin Invest 1993;92:503−508.
6. Petkau A, Chelack WS. Radioprotective effect of SOD on model phospholipid membrane. Biochim Biophys Acta 1988;433:445−456.
7. Quintiliani M. The oxygen effect in radiation interaction on DNA and enzymes. Int J Radiat Biol 1986;50:573−594.
8. Otero G, Avila MA, Emfietzoglou D, Clerch LB, Massaro D, Notario V. Increased manganese superoxide dismutase activity, protein, and mRNA levels and concurrent induction of tumor necrosis factor alpha in radiation-initiated Syrian hamster cells. Molec Carcinogenesis 1996; 17:175−180.
9. Akashi M, Hachiya M, Paquette RL, Osawa Y, Shimizu S, Susuki G. Irradiation increases manganese superoxide dismutase mRNA levels in human fibroblast. Possible mechanism for its accumulation. J Biol Chem 1995;30:15864−15869.
10. Yamaoka K, Edamatsu M, Mori A. Increased SOD activity and decreased lipid peroxide levels induced by low dose X-irradiation in rat organs. Free Radic Biol Med 1991;11:299−306.
11. Meister A, Anderson ME. Glutathione. Ann Rev Biochem 1983;52:711−760.
12. Meister A. Metabolism and fuction of glutathione. In: Dolphin D, Poulson R, Avramovic O (eds) Glutathione: Chemical, Biochemical and Medical Aspects. New York: Wiley 1989; 367−474.
13. Anderson ME. Glutathione and glutathione delivery compounds. Adv Pharmacol 1997;38: 65−78.
14. Kojima S, Matsuki O, Kinoshita I, Gonzalez-Valdes T, Shimura N, Kubodera A. Does small-dose γ-ray radiation induce endogenous antioxidant potential in vivo? Biol Pharm Bull 1997;20:601−604.
15. Kojima S, Matsuki O, Nomura T, Kubodera A, Yamaoka K. Elevation of mouse liver glutathione level by low-dose γ-ray irradiation and its effect on CCl_4-induced liver damage. Anticancer Res 1998;18:2471−2476.
16. Kojima S, Matsuki O, Nomura T, Kubodera A, Honda Y, Honda S, Tanooka H, Wakasugi H, Yamaoka K. Induction of mRNAs for glutathione-related proteins in mouse liver by low doses of γ-rays. Biochim Biophys Acta 1998;1381:312−318.
17. Kojima S, Matsuki O, Nomura T, Shimura N, Kubodera A, Yamaoka K, Tanooka H, Wakasugi H, Honda Y, Honda S, Sasaki T. Localization of glutathione and induction glutathione synthesis-related proteins in mouse brain by low doses of γ-rays. Brain Res 1998;808:262−269.
18. Kojima S, Matsuki O, Nomura T, Yamaoka K, Takayashi M, Niki E. Elevation of antioxidant potency in the brain of mice by low-dose γ-ray irradiation and its effect on 1-methyl-4-phenyl-1,2,3,6-tetrahydropyridine (MPTP)-induced brain damage. Free Radic Biol Med 1999;26: 388−395.

19. Xia E, Rao GF, Remmen H, Heydari AR, Richardson A. Activities of antioxidant enzymes in various tissues of male Fischer 344 rats are altered by food restriction. J Nutr 1995;125: 195—201.
20. Sedlack J, Lindsay RH. Estimation of total protein-bound and nonprotein sulfhydryl group in tissue with Ellman's reagent. Anal Biochem 1968;25:192—205.
21. Lowry O, Rosebrough N, Farr L, Randall RJ. Protein measurement with the Folin phenol reagent. J Biol Chem 1951;183:265—275.
22. Moore WR, Anderson ME, Meister A, Murata K, Kimura A. Increased capacity for glutathione synthesis enhances resistance to radiation in Escherichia coli: a possible model for mammalian cell protection. Proc Natl Acad Sci USA 1989;86:1461—1464.
23. Beutler E. Effect of flavin compounds on glutathione reductase activity: in vivo and in vitro studies. J Clin Invest 1969;48:1957—1966.
24. Kitaoka Y, Sorachi K, Nakamura H, Masutani H, Mitsui A, Kobayashi F, Mori T, Yodoi J. Detection of adult T cell leukemia-derived factor (ADF)/human thioredoxin in human serum. Immunol Lett 1994;42:155—161.
25. Luthman M, Holmgren A. Rat liver thioredoxin and thioredoxin reductase: purification and characterization. Biochem 1982;21:6628—6633.
26. Iwata S, Hori T, Sato N, Ueda-Taniguchi Y, Yamabe T, Nakamura H, Masutani H, Yodoi J. Thiol-mediated redox regulation of lymphocyte proliferation. J Immunol 1994;152:5633—5642.
27. Prasad AV, Mohan N, Chadrasekar B, Meltz L. Induction of "immediately early genes" by low-dose ionizing radiation. Radiat Res 1995;143:263—272.
28. Okamoto T, Ogiwara H, Hayashi T, Mitsui A, Kawabe T, Yodoi J. Human thioredoxin/adult T cell leukemia-derived factor activates the enhancer binding protein of human immunodeficiency virus type I by thiol redox control mechanism. Int Immunol 1992;4:811—819.
29. Schenk HM, Klein W, Erdbrügger W, Dröge W, Schulze-Osthoff K. Distinct effects of thioredoxin and antioxidants on the activation of transcription factors NF-kappa B and AP-1. Proc Natl Acad Sci USA 1994;91:1672—1676.
30. Xanthoudakis S, Miao G, Pan YC, Curran T. Redox activation of Fos-Jun DNA binding activity is mediated by a DNA repair enzyme. EMBO J 1992;11:3323—3335.
31. Meyer M, Schreck R, Baeuerle PA. H_2O_2 and antioxidants have opposite effects on activation of NF-κB and AP-1 in intact cells: AP-1 as secondary antioxidant-responsive factor. EMBO J 1993;12:2005—2015.

On mechanistic studies of immune responses following low-dose ionizing radiation

Shu-Zheng Liu and Ou Bai

MH Radiobiology Research Unit, Norman Bethune University of Medical Sciences, Changchun, China

Abstract. The present paper reviews the low-dose radiation (LDR)-induced intercellular reactions in the immune organs and their molecular basis. There exist delicate interactions between the lymphocytes and the accessory cells by direct contact via surface molecules as well as by paracrine and autocrine action via secretion of cytokines and growth factors. These events were found to be activated after LDR. The multiple signal transduction pathways activated in the immune cells led to positive and negative regulation of cellular processes forming a complex signal transduction network. Whole-body irradiation (WBI) with low-dose X-rays caused facilitation of these pathways with enhanced expression or increased activity of some important signal molecules and suppression of others leading to induction of genes related to lymphocyte survival and proliferation. The present state of knowledge indicates that more work has to be done on the effect of different doses of ionizing radiation on these regulatory mechanisms within the immune system. It is emphasized that in a complex organism there exist defense and adaptive mechanisms at the molecular and cellular (as well as systemic) levels which produce a response to ionizing radiation, and these have to be considered as a whole in mechanistic studies of the biological effects of low level exposures.

Keywords: genetic regulation, immune system, intercellular reactions, low-dose radiation, signal transduction.

Introduction

The immune system is one of the most important constituent parts of the mammalian defense mechanisms guarding the body against infection and cancer. Most carcinogens are immunosuppressants. Ionizing radiation at medium to high doses is known to be carcinogenic and to induce suppression of the immune system. However, low-level radiation may have different effects. Epidemiological and radiobiological studies have demonstrated that low-level radiation may not increase the cancer risk, and it has been observed to decrease the excess relative risk of cancer in the 40—70 years age group in a high background radiation area (HBRA) with an exposure rate 3.6 times as high as that of the control [1]. The immune responses have been found to be upregulated in the inhabitants in this HBRA. It has also been demonstrated in experimental animals that WBI with low-dose X- and γ-rays stimulates immunity [2—4]. It was recently observed that pre-exposure of C57BL/6J mice with LDR has been found to decrease the

Address for correspondence: Prof Shu-Zheng Liu, MH Radiobiology Research Unit, Norman Bethune University of Medical Sciences, 8 Xinmin Street, Changchun 130021, China. Tel.: +86-431-567-6947. Fax: +86-431-563-3205. E-mail: szl@public.cc.jl.cn

rate of occurrence of thymic lymphoma induced by split-dose (1.75 Gy once a week for 4 consecutive weeks) irradiation and this effect was accompanied with an enhancing action of LDR on immunity [5]. Therefore, elucidation of the mechanisms of the upregulation of immune responses to LDR may shed light on the nature of hormesis with low-level exposures. To do this, radiobiologists have to follow closely the rapid progress in the studies on immune regulation. Firstly, recent studies have demonstrated the delicate interactions between the lymphocytes and the accessory cells by direct contact via surface molecules and by paracrine and/or autocrine action via cytokines and growth factors. Secondly, the multiple signal pathways of the immune cells activated by external and internal stimuli have been gradually disclosed, demonstrating positive and negative regulation within the cells forming a complex signal transduction network. Thirdly, the molecular regulation of cell survival and death, as well as maturation, differentiation, and activation, has been found to be important in the understanding of the immune response (to different agents) from both the internal and external environment. The three aspects are intimately interconnected, and a separate discussion of each of them is only to be given for convenience. In the following sections a brief account of what has been studied and what remains to be elucidated will be outlined.

Interactions between T lymphocytes and accessory cells

It has been repeatedly observed that LDR stimulates the reactivity of peripheral blood and splenic lymphocytes to PHA and Con A [2—4] and that spontaneous incorporation of ^{3}H-TdR into thymocytes is markedly increased after WBI with low doses [6]. It implicates that both the central and peripheral compartments of the T cell system are involved in LDR-induced stimulation. Upregulated reactivity of T cells to mitogens would lead to increased induction and secretion of a series of cytokines initiating interactions among the cells in the immune system. The increased secretion of CSF (GM-CSF and G-CSF, etc.) by thymocytes after LDR would lead to maturation and proliferation of macrophages and granulocytes [7]. These phagocytic cells play an important role in innate immunity by engulfing and destroying foreign cells. The antigen-presenting cells (APCs), including macrophages and dendritic cells, are of special importance in their dual functions by presenting specific as well as nonspecific signals leading to activation of the helper and cytotoxic T cells (T_H and T_C) in the presence of co-stimulating signal molecules. At the same time the APCs also secret IL-12, IL-1β, TNFα, and others that modulate the activity of the lymphocytes via corresponding receptors as well as providing autocrine functions to the APCs themselves. LDR stimulates the induction of IL-12, IL-1β and TNFα in the macrophages. The production of NO by, and expression of iNOS (inducible NO synthase) in macrophages was upregulated after LDR (Sun and Liu, in press). It is known that TNFα and IL-1β may facilitate the nuclear translocation of NF-κB partly via NO and ROIs (reactive oxygen intermediates). The recently reported reciprocal control of helper T cell and dendritic cell differentiation has shed light on the delicate interrelations between these cells [8]. Studies on the possible differential radiosensitivity between dendritic cell subsets would further elucidate the mechanism.

Involvement of multiple signal transduction pathways

The signal transduction system in a typical eukaryotic cell consists of a network of proteins that transform multiple external stimuli into appropriate cellular responses. Macromolecular organization is important in signal transduction. It is known now that molecules that form this network can be placed into ordered biochemical pathways in which signal propagation occurs through the sequential establishment of protein-protein and small molecule-protein interactions.

It has been demonstrated that T cell activation by LDR involves the facilitation of signal transduction initiated in the TCR/CD3 complex and G protein/adenylate cyclase system [9—11]. WBI of mice with low-dose X-rays caused increased expression of TCR and CD3 molecules on the thymocytes leading to mobilization of $[Ca^{2+}]_i$ and activation of PKCα, β_1 and β_2, followed by upregulated transcription of c-fos and bcl-2 as well as increased expression of Fos and Bcl-2 proteins. It was found that the upregulation of CD3, $[Ca^{2+}]_i$ and calcineurin showed a similar time course after WBI with 0.075 Gy. These changes would lead to activation of the transcription factors such as NF-κB important in the induction of the cytokine genes and survival genes [12]. A significant decrease in cAMP and increase in cGMP with marked lowering of cAMP/cGMP ratio as well as downregulation of the PKA activity in the thymocytes were found after LDR, suggesting the involvement of G protein/adenylate cyclase system in the activation of T cells. PLA$_2$ activity was lowered after LDR that would lead to decreased production of the immunosuppressor PGE$_2$ which also lowers the activity of PKA. It was recently reported that phosphodiesterase-7 (PDE7) induction accompanying CD3 and CD28 costimulation with consequent decrease of cAMP and suppression of PKA activity is required for T cell activation [13]. This gives support to our observation that the cAMP pathway is involved in LDR-induced activation of the thymocytes. It remains to be disclosed whether other signal pathways, including those related to hormonal changes, e.g., the hypothalamus-pituitary-adrenocortical system, are also involved [14—17]. A schematic diagram is presented in Fig. 1 to show the interrelation of the chief signal pathways activated after LDR and their relation to the intercellular changes. In this diagram the intercellular changes induced by low-dose radiation include the reaction between the APCs (represented by macrophages) and the T cells. LDR enhances the secretion of IL-12, IL-1β and TNFα which act on the T cells via related receptors to influence the maturation, differentiation, and activation of the T cells. LDR may also increase the expression of the surface molecules such as B7-1/2 and MHC I/II of the APCs, thus enhancing the intercellular reactions (unpublished data, not shown in the diagram). On the left side of the

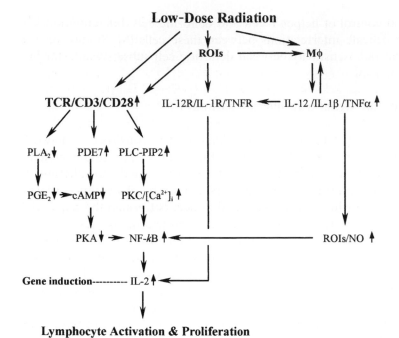

Lymphocyte Activation & Proliferation

Fig. 1. Schematic diagram of the interrelationship of the chief signal pathways related to the activation of immune responses after low-dose radiation. ROI = reactive oxygen intermediate; Mφ = macrophage; TCR = T cell receptor; IL = interleukin; TNF = tumor necrosis factor; R = receptor; PLA = phospholipase A; PDE = phosphodiesterase; PLC = phospholipase C; PIP2 = phosphatidylinositol biphosphate; PGE = prostaglandin E; cAMP = cyclic adenosine monophosphate; PKC = protein kinase C; $[Ca^{2+}]_i$ = intracellular concentration of free calcium ions; PKA = protein kinase A; NO = nitric oxide; NF-κB = nuclear factor kappaB. See text for detailed explanations.

diagram three signal pathways are displayed to show their interrelations with the result of facilitation of nuclear translocation of NF-κB which would cause induction of a series of genes related to cellular activation [9,18,19]. In the diagram only IL-2 is shown as a representative. Others are discussed in the next paragraph. On the right side of the diagram it is shown that IL-1β and TNFα may also facilitate the nuclear translocation of NF-κB via ROIs and/or NO [20].

Molecular changes related to cell survival and proliferation

It is well known that the lymphoid tissue is one of the most radiosensitive constituents of the body and lymphocytes would undergo apoptosis after exposure to a moderate dose of ionizing radiation. However, it has been demonstrated in mice that the dose-effect relationship of thymocyte apoptosis 12−24 h after WBI presents a J-shaped curve with the apoptotic rate decreasing to below control level after doses within 0.1 Gy [11,18]. Mechanistic studies disclosed that the genes and their protein products related to cell survival and death responded differently to different doses of radiation. For example, WBI with 0.075 Gy caused prompt upregulation of c-fos and bcl-2 transcription within 1 h, followed by increased expression of c-Fos and Bcl-2 proteins within 8 and 12 h, respectively, in the thymus, while WBI with 2 Gy led to an opposite effect. Molecules facilitating apoptosis, including ICE, Bad, p53, Rb, Fas ligand, and Gadd45 were found to be downregulated at mRNA and/or protein level after WBI with 0.075 Gy and upregulated after WBI with 2 Gy. A time course study of the apoptotic rate by an in situ end-labeling assay in frozen sections of the thymus showed different time course of changes after different doses. At doses of 0.05 and 0.075 Gy an abrupt increase of apoptotic rate was followed by a drop to below control level at 12 h. At the dose of 0.025 Gy this early increase was slight and not followed by a significant decrease. A dose of 2 Gy caused sustained increase of apoptotic rate in much greater amplitude followed by a decrease only after 72 h. This observation might implicate:

1) the damage caused by 0.05 and 0.075 Gy would stimulate the biological control system;
2) the slight damage caused by 0.025 Gy was not enough to arouse such a response; and
3) and the huge damage caused by 2 Gy would have over-saturated the control mechanism with its recovery only after 72 h.

Recent studies have disclosed that the TNF-receptor-associated factors (TRAFs) form a family of cytoplasmic adaptor proteins that mediate signal transduction from many members of the TNFR (tumor necrosis factor receptor) superfamily and IL-1R (interleukin-1 receptor) [20]. They are important in the regulation of cell survival and proliferation. LDR-induced increase in IL-1β and TNFα secretion by the APCs would act via the receptors to activate the MAPKK adaptor protein TAK1 that associates with TRAF2/6 to form cIAP (cellular inhibitor of apoptosis), a signal upstream of NIK (NF-κB inducing kinase). Activation of NIK would lead to stimulation of IKK (IκB kinase) resulting in phosphorylation and ubiquitation of IκB with the final outcome of translocation of NF-κB into the nucleus. The latter binds to genes related to survival and proliferation of the lymphocytes [21]. TNFα and IL-1β also exert profound influence on the maturation and function of APCs themselves [22]. During the first 24 h after stimulation with LPS or TNFα, up to 10^6 molecules of class II MHC are deposited on the cell surface, arising from both redistribution and de novo synthesis. Judging from these molecular changes it can be anticipated that an increase of secretion of IL-1β and TNFα following LDR would have a profound influence on the immune status of the organism.

The Bcl-2/Bax ratio and Bcl-X$_L$/Bad ratio in the thymocytes were found to be raised after LDR, being important factors promoting cell survival (Liu et al., in press). It has been documented that Ca^{2+}-triggered signaling cascade may promote cell survival through the calmodulin-dependent protein kinase (kinase that activates protein kinase B) resulting in phosphorylation of Bad on serine residue 136 and inhibition of apoptosis [19]. This action of Ca^{2+} may also be related to the upregulation of calcineurin that is a protein phosphatase down-stream of calmodulin and related to translocation of NF-κB into the nucleus facilitating cell survival, as shown in a previous section of the present paper.

The molecules of the caspase (cystein-containing aspartate-specific protease) family are closely related to regulation of cell survival and death. Caspase-3 occupies an important position in this network. The action of these molecules is antagonized by other factors. It has recently been found that a new inhibitor of apoptosis (IAP) protein named survivin, normally expressed in the G_2/M phase of the cell cycle, is associated with microtubules of the mitotic spindle. Disruption of the survivin-microtubule interactions results in loss of the anti-apoptotic function of survivin and increased caspase-3 activity [23]. All these data would give important initiatives for further studies on the mechanism of the above mentioned characteristic features of apoptosis in the immune system after LDR.

Conclusion

The above brief comments hint at a number of points. First of all, the complexity of the immune system and the regulation of the immune responses (as gradually disclosed in recent years) calls for close attention of radiobiologists to more basic studies in this field in order to cope with the rapidly accumulating data for the design of mechanistic studies. The second point to be mentioned is the necessity of viewing the organism as a whole in the studies of the effects of low-dose radiation. There are changes caused by low-dose radiation that cannot be analyzed by DNA damage alone. The last, but not the least important, is the correlation of the changes observed at the different levels of the hierarchically organized systems in the body to fully understand the meaning and significance of the phenomena observed at each level. To accomplish such studies collaborative research is needed.

Acknowledgements

This work was supported by grants from NSFC.

References

1. Wei L-X, Wang J-Z. Estimate of cancer risk for a population continuously exposed to higher background radiation in Yangjiang, China. Int J Occup Med Toxicol 1994;3:195–201.
2. Liu SZ. Current status of research on radiation hormesis in the immune system after low level radiation. J Radiat Res Radiat Proces 1995;13:129–139.
3. James SJ, Makinodan T. T cell proliferation in normal and autoimmune-prone mice after extended exposure to low doses of ionizing radiation and/or caloric restriction. Int J Radiat Biol 1988;53:137–152.
4. Hattori S. State of research and perspective on radiation hormesis in Japan. Int J Occup Med Toxicol 1994;3:203–217.
5. Li XY, Li XJ, Zhang Y, Lu Z, Liu SZ. The effect of low dose ionizing radiation on thymic lym-

phoma induced in mice by carcinogenic dose of radiation. Chin Acad Periodical Abst 1998;4:1406—1407.

6. Liu Shu-Zheng. Cellular basis of immunoenhancement following low dose radiation. Proceedings of China-Japan Medical Conference Beijing, China. 1992;100—104.

7. Zhang HL, Zhang M, Liu SZ. Effect of low dose X-irradiation on CSF secretion of mouse lung cells, thymocytes and splenocytes. Chin J Radiol Med Prot 1992;12:162—165.

8. Rissoan M-C, Soumelis V, Kadowaki N, Grouard G, Briere F, Malefy R, de W, Liu Y-J. Reciprocal control of T helper cell and dendritic cell differentiation. Science 1999;283:1183—1186.

9. Liu SZ, Su X, Zhang YC, Zhao Y. Signal transduction in lymphocytes after low dose radiation. Int J Occup Med Toxicol 1994;3:107—117.

10. Liu SZ. Cellular and molecular basis of the stimulatory effect of low dose radiation on immunity. In: Wei LX, Sugahara T, Tao ZF (eds) High Levels of Natural Radiation. Amsterdam: Elsevier Science BV, 1997;341—353.

11. Liu SZ. Biological defense and adaptation induced by low dose radiation. Human and ecological risk assessment (HERA) 1998;4:1217—1254.

12. Chen SL, Liu SZ. Activation of transcription factor CREB and NF-κB in murine immune cells after WBI with 75mGy X-rays. J Radiat Res Radiat Proces 1998;16:45—49.

13. Li L, Yee C, Beavo JA. CD3- and CD28-dependent induction of PDE7 required for T cell activation. Science 1999;283:848—851.

14. Ulloa L, Doody J, Massague J. Inhibition of transforming growth factor-/SMAD signaling by the interferon-γ/STAT pathway. Nature 1999;397:710—712.

15. Seder RA, Marth T, Sieve MC, Strober W, Letterio JJ, Roberts AB, Kelsall B. Factors involved in the differentiation of TGF-β-producing cells from naive CD4$^+$ T cells: IL-4 and IFN-γ have opposing effects, while TGF-β positively regulates its own production. J Immunol 1998;160: 5719—5728.

16. Groux H, O'Garra A, Bigler M, Rouleau M, Antonenko S, de Vries JE, Roncarolo MG. A CD4$^+$ T-cell subset inhibits antigen-specific T-cell responses and prevents colitis. Nature 1997;389: 737—742.

17. Liu SZ, Zhao Y, Han ZB, Gong SL, Zhang M, Liu WH. Role of changes in functional status of hypothamic-pituitary-adrenocortical axis in immunoenbancement after low dose radiation. Chin J Radiol Med Prot 1994;14:11—14.

18. Liu SZ, Zhang YC, Mu Y, Su X, Liu JX. Thymocyte apoptosis in response to low dose radiation. Mutat Res 1996;58:185—191.

19. Yano S, Tokumitsu R, Soderling TR. Calcium promotes cell survival through CaM-K kinase activation of the protein-kinase-B pathway. Nature 1998;396:584—586.

20. Ninomiya-Tsuji J, Kishimoto K, Hiyama A, Inoue J, Cao Z, Matsumoto K. The kinase TAK1 can activate the NIK-I-kappaB as well as the MAP kinase cascade in the IL-1 signaling pathway. Nature 1999;398:252—254.

21. Ashkenazi A, Dixit VM. Death receptors: signaling and modulation. Science 1998;281: 1305—1308.

22. Marina C, Engering A, Pinet V, Pieters J, Lanzavecchia A. Inflammatory stimuli induce accumulation of MHC class II complexes on dendritic cells. Nature 1997;388:782—787.

23. Li F, Ambrosini G, Chu EY, Plescia J, Tognin S, Maarchisio CP, Altieri DC. Control of apoptosis and mitotic spindle checkpoint by survivin. Nature 1998;396:580—583.

Cancer and epidemiology

Concerted DNA repair and apoptosis responsible for threshold effects in radiation risk

Sohei Kondo

Atomic Energy Research Institute, Kinki University, Higashiosaka, Japan

Abstract. The major risks of low-dose radiation are mutagenesis, teratogenesis, and carcinogenesis. All three have been shown (experimentally) to approach zero risk with decreasing dose rate, demonstrating the critical contribution of DNA repair at low dose-rate irradiation. However, DNA repair is not perfect. There must be defense mechanisms other than DNA repair. In p53(–/–) mouse embryos, radiation remains teratogenic even when given at a very low dose-rate, this is because p53(–/–) mouse embryos are unable to carry out apoptosis. Multiple lines of evidence are given to support the hypothesis that when DNA-repair functions efficiently in concerted cooperation with vigorous p53-dependent apoptosis, there is a threshold dose-rate for induction of malformation (or thymic lymphoma) by radiation in mice.

Keywords: antiapoptosis, lifetime β-irradiation, p53-dependent apoptosis, thymic lymphoma, tumor promoter.

Concerted DNA repair and apoptosis responsible for complete elimination of teratogenic damage after irradiation

For p53(+/+) mice with the wild-type p53 gene, acute (0.45 Gy/min) X-irradiation of embryos at E9.5 (embryonic age of 9.5 days) with 2 Gy was highly lethal (60% deaths) and considerably teratogenic (50% anomalies) whereas for p53(–/–) mice with a deficient p53 gene, the same treatment was only slightly lethal (7% deaths) but highly teratogenic (80% anomalies) [1,2]. Frequency of cells dying by apoptosis after irradiation at E9.5 with 2 Gy markedly increased (60%) for p53(+/+) embryos but did not increase for p53(–/–) embryos [1,2]. However, when the dose of 2 Gy was given at the same E9.5 but at a 400-fold lower dose-rate (1.2 mGy/min), the dose was no longer teratogenic for p53(+/+) embryos which are capable of p53-dependent apoptosis, whereas it remained teratogenic for p53(–/–) embryos unable to carry out apoptosis [3; F. Kato, personal communication].

Hence, complete elimination of teratogenic damage from irradiated tissues requires a concerted cooperation of two independent functions: proficient DNA repair, which occurs under chronic irradiation conditions [3], and competent apoptosis, which is specific to midgestational embryos [2,3].

Address for correspondence: Prof Sohei Kondo, Atomic Energy Research Institute, Kinki University, Higashiosaka 577-8502, Japan. Tel.: +81-729-562576. Fax: +81-729-562576.
E-mail: skondo@taurus.bekkoame.ne.jp

Dose-rate dependence of radiation mutagenesis in mice

Mutation frequency F (locus^{-1}) at coat color loci of mice increases linearly with radiation dose D (Gy) as follows:

$$F = a + mD \tag{1}$$

where a is the spontaneous mutation rate and m the induced mutation rate (Gy^{-1}). For spermatogonia [4]:

$$m = 2(\pm 0.4) \times 10^{-5} (at\ 0.9\ Gy/min)\ or\ 0.7\ (\pm 0.2) \times 10^{-5} (at\ 8 \sim 0.007\ mGy/min) \tag{2}$$

For oocytes [5],

$$m = 1 \sim 4 \times 10^{-5} (at\ 0.9\ Gy/min)\ or\ 0\ (for\ 4\ Gy\ at\ 0.09\ mGy/min) \tag{3}$$

Apoptosis induction in thymus of mice after whole body irradiation [6]

After whole body X-irradiation of mice, frequency P of apoptotic lymphocytes in the thymus increased linearly with dose D (Gy) as follows:

$$P = P_o + bD;\ b = 0.18\ (Gy^{-1})\ after\ acute\ (0.3\ Gy/min)\ irradiation \tag{4}$$

where P is measured 4 h after irradiation, P_o is the spontaneous P value and b the rate per Gy of induced apoptotic frequency. The P value reaches a maximum 4 h after irradiation.

The thymus weight W and the total number N of lymphocytes in the thymus, both measured 24 h postirradiation, decreased approximately as follows:

$$(W - W_r) = (W_o - W_r)\ exp\ (-wD);\ w = 0.43(Gy^{-1})\ after\ acute\ (0.3\ Gy/min)\ irradiation \tag{5}$$

$$N/N_o = S = exp\ (-kD);\ k = 1.1\ (Gy^1)\ after\ irradiation\ at\ 3\ or\ 0.003\ Gy/min \tag{6}$$

where W_r is the weight of the apoptosis-resistant fraction of the thymus, W_o the W value before irradiation, w the rate per Gy of radiation-induced reduction in W; N_o is the N value before irradiation, S is survival and k the rate per Gy of radiation-induced reduction in survival S.

As seen in Equations (5) and (6), thymus atrophy was observed 24 h after irradiation. The shrinkage in the size of the thymus (as indicated by both parameters) is the end result of the total apoptotic cell deaths that occurred in the organ one to several hours after irradiation. As shown in Equation (6), the rate per Gy of the total apoptotic deaths in lymphocytes by 24 h postirradiation is independent of the dose-rate. This indicates that apoptotic lymphocyte death occurs so promptly that the relatively slow processes of DNA repair (of radiation-induced double-strand breaks in DNA [3]) does not affect the rate of apoptosis.

It is intriguing that the k value given in Equation (6) is accurate only when D is close to 1 Gy; it decreases with increase in D. This indicates that susceptibility to apoptosis decreases with an increase in the dose of radiation (in spite of the fact that apoptotic frequency P increases linearly with D in the range up to 4 Gy, see Equation (4)). These results indicate that while the majority of lymphocytes show prompt apoptotic responses to radiation, there is a fraction of surviving lymphocytes that show antiapoptotic responses, undergoing growth arrest. These variations in cellular responses probably reflect variations in p53 protein levels in lymphocytes. Only the cells with high p53 protein levels may commit prompt apoptosis.

As seen in Table 1, after X-irradiation with 2 Gy, the weight of the p53(+/+) thymus decreased from 55 to 32 mg 24 h postirradiation and remained at the same reduced weight until 72 h, indicating that the surviving T cells were at growth arrest during the 24 to 72 h period. By contrast, in p53(−/−) mice, the weight of the thymus increased 24 h after irradiation from 71 to 78 mg with a concomitant increase in the lymphocyte content by 70%, showing that radiation can induce hypertrophy in p53(−/−) thymuses unable to carry out apoptosis.

Threshold dose-rate for induction of thymic lymphoma in mice after internal whole-body irradiation with tritium β-rays

Yamamoto et al. [7,8] administered drinking water containing tritium at various concentrations to mice for a lifetime. Resultant lymphoma incidences in the thymus are plotted in Fig. 1 against the logarithm of the dose-rate of internal β-rays from the administered tritiated drinking water. As seen from the incidence vs. dose-rate curve in Fig. 1, the lymphoma incidence F_{lym} versus dose-rate dD/dt (cGy/day) relationship can be classified into four parts as follows:

1   In the high dose-rate range, 9.6–24 cGy/day,

$$F_{lym} = 0.54 + 0.004 dD/dt \qquad (7)$$

Table 1. Change in the weight and the lymphocyte content of the thymus after acute X-irradiation (from [6]).

Genotype of mice	Dose (Gy)	Time after irradiation	Weight (mg)	Lymphocyte content (10^6 cells)
p52(+/+)	0	0 h	55	147
	2	24 h	32	33
	2	72 h	32	NT[a]
p53(−/−)	0	0 h	71	147
	2	24 h	78	242
	2	72 h	69	NT[a]

[a]NT = Not tested.

2. In the intermediate dose rate range, 2.4—9.6 cGy/day,

$$F_{lym} = 0.05 + 0.07 dD/dt \qquad (8)$$

3. In the low dose-rate range, 0.4—2.4 cGy/day,

$$F_{lym} = 0.046 + 0.01 dD/dt \qquad (9)$$

4. In the extremely low dose-rate range, 0.02—0.09 cGy/day,

$$F_{lym} = 0 \qquad (10)$$

As seen from Equations (7) to (10), lifetime whole-body internal β-irradiation is not tumorigenic in the lowest dose-rate range (0.02—0.09 cGy/day), slightly tumorigenic in the low dose-rate range (0.4—2.4 cGy/day) and highly tumorigenic in the intermediate dose-rate range (2.4—9.6 cGy/day). In the high dose-rate range, 9.6—24 cGy/day, the tumorigenicity of β-rays begins to plateau.

Radiation is the promoter for thymic lymphoma development in mice

Saccharin is not a mutagen but it induces bladder cancer in rats after lifetime dietary administration at high doses; it stimulates proliferation of target cells responsible for production of bladder cancer, whereas, at low doses, it does not induce bladder cancer, i.e., it has a no-effect threshold [9].
   A no-effect threshold was also observed for the relation of the thymic lymphoma incidence in mice to the dose-rate of internal β-rays from the tritiated drinking water administered for a lifetime (Fig. 1). This means that the administered

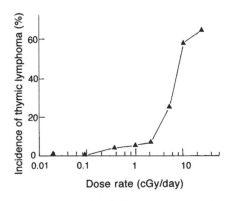

Fig. 1. Incidence of thymic lymphoma in mice plotted against the dose-rate of internal β-irradiation. Female mice were given drinking water containing different concentrations of tritium for a lifetime. The levels of tritium consumed by mice are expressed in terms of rates of internal β-ray doses averaged over the whole body. (Modified from Yamamoto et al. [7,8].)

tritium β-radiation cannot be the mutagenic initiator for induction of lymphoma in mice because in general, frequency of mutations is very low and it increases linearly with radiation dose without threshold (Equations (1) to (3)). Therefore, we assume that β-radiation given by tritium administration acts as a tumor promoter.

In Fig. 2, cumulative thymic lymphoma incidences are plotted against the age of mice for different levels of the ß-irradiation dose-rate/the total lifetime dose. As seen from the three curves for dose-rates of 24, 9.6 and 4.8 cGy/day, the total number of lymphomas in each group appeared at the mean ages of 34, 52, and 72 weeks, respectively (that is, at mean latency periods of 24, 42, and 62 weeks after the start of the β-irradiation, respectively). It should be noted that the maximum variation within each of the mean latency periods is only 10 to 14 weeks for the three groups. If the radiation-induced tumorigenesis results from stochastic events during lifetime irradiation, we expect much wider variation in the mean latent period than 10 to 14 weeks. We may conclude that thymic lymphomas are produced as a result of deterministic events, probably radiation-induced tissue injury (see below).

I proposed the tissue-repair error model for radiation caricnogenesis; tumors result from promoting effects of a growth stimulating milieu created for repair of injury induced by radiation [10,11]. This wound-healing error model is supported by the following findings: for rats after weaning, saccharin is carcinogenic when given after the epithelium has been ulcerated by freezing, whereas without the freezing treatment it is not carcinogenic [9]. Incidentally, we found that if thymic lymphocytes have a defective p53 gene, they show positive responses to growth stimulating factors induced by radiation (Table 1). In contrast, normal p53(+/+) thymic lymphocytes do not respond to the radiation-induced growth stimulating factors; they commit apoptosis or undergo growth arrest in response to radiation (see Equation (4) and Table 1). Therefore, if there had existed "spon-

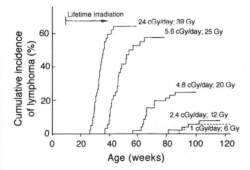

Fig. 2. Cumulative incidences of thymic lymphoma plotted against the age of mice for different β-irradiation dose rates. Female mice were given drinking water containing different concentrations of tritium for a lifetime. The levels of administered tritium are expressed in terms of the rate of internal β-ray dose averaged over the whole body; the dose-rates and the total lifetime doses are denoted beside each cumulative incidence curve. From S. Yamamoto (personal communication).

taneous" prelymphoma-type cells with a defective p53 gene [12] in the thymus of mice when β-irradiation was started, those p53(–/–) pretumorous cells would have responded positively to growth stimulating factors produced by radiation, thus resulting in radiation-induced clonal expansion of the pretumorous cells (see [12] in the case of tumor cells). In support of the above-mentioned speculation, spontaneous lymphoma incidence in p53(–/–) mice increases rapidly from 15 weeks of age and reaches 100% at 27 weeks, whereas 4 Gy given at 6 days of age shortens the latency period for lymphoma development by 10 weeks [13] (see [11] for more detailed discussion). These results support the notion that radiation acts as the tumor promoter for production of thymic lymphoma when the radiation level is higher than the threshold for induction of tissue damage in the thymus.

Threshold for radiation induction of tumor promoting activity

We assume that the activity of the radiation-induced tumor promoters Q (μm) is proportional to dose-rate dD/dt in the case of lifetime irradiation as follows:

$$Q = Q_o + \alpha dD/dt \quad (11)$$

where Q_o is a dose-rate independent component and α is a proportionality coefficient.

The tumor promoter model of radiation for lymphoma implies that lymphoma frequency F_{lym} is proportional to Q as follows:

$$F_{lym} = cQ = cQ_o + c\alpha dD/dt \tag{12}$$

where c is a constant of proportionality.

Comparing Equation (12) with Equations (7) and (10), we reach the following conclusions. The α value is large (0.07) in the dose-rate range of 2.4–9.6 cGy/day whereas α is small (0.01) in the dose-rate range of 0.4–2.4 cGy/day. This indicates that 2.4 cGy/day could be close to the threshold dose-rate below which tumor promoter activity is not induced by radiation. Equation (12) is not applicable to Equation (7) as its constant term is markedly different from those in Equations (8) and (9).

Threshold dose-rate for radiation induction of antiapoptosis activity

At 1 cGy/day, which is below 2.4 cGy/day (the threshold dose-rate for tumor promoter induction), β-irradiation is still tumorigenic, yielding 6% thymic lymphomas (Fig. 2). These lymphomas appeared at the age of 100 weeks, that is, after a long latency period of 90 weeks (Fig. 2). How can the radiation-induced tumorigenic effect be remembered for such a long time by target cells that will later develop into tumor cells? It is tempting to assume that after the start of irradiation, a fraction of irradiated thymic lymphocytes, which happen to retain un-repaired DNA damage, does not commit apoptosis but undergoes growth arrest for a long time without developing into maturation, i.e., remaining as primordial cells due to enhanced expression of p21 [14]. Such primordial cells could be responsible for production of lymphomas a long time after the start of lifetime β-irradiation at 1 cGy/day.

In contrast, lifetime β-irradiation at the extremely low dose-rate of 0.09 or 0.02 cGy/day is not tumorigenic. This indicates that the dose-rate of about 0.1 cGy/day is the threshold below which irradiation does not induce antiapoptotic activity but induces only proapoptotic activity in lymphocytes (so that if cells retain unrepaired DNA damage, they are completely eliminated from irradiated tissues by apoptosis), thus ensuring the zero risk of radiation below the threshold.

Acknowledgements

I am grateful to T. Norimura, F. Kato, O. Yamamoto and K. Fujikawa for the information on unpublished data; and to K.S. Iwamoto and H. Ryo for comments and suggestions during preparation of the manuscript.

References

1. Norimura T, Nomoto S, Katsuki M, Gondo Y, Kondo S. p53-dependent apoptosis suppresses radiation-induced teratogenesis. Nat Med 1996;2:577—580.
2. Nomoto S, Ootsuyama A, Shioyama Y, Katsuki M, Kondo S, Norimura T. The high susceptibility of heterozygous p53(+/−) mice to malformation after foetal irradiation is related to sub-comptent apoptosis. Int J Radiat Biol 1998;74:419—429.
3. Kondo S. Threshold effects in radiation risk arising from concerted DNA repair and apoptosis. Radiat Res (In press).
4. Russell WL, Kelly EM. Mutation frequencies in male mice and the estimation of genetic hazards of radiation in men. Proc Natl Acad Sci USA 1982;79:542—544.
5. Russell WL. Mutation frequencies in female mice and estimation of genetic hazards of radiation in women. Proc Natl Acad Sci USA 1977;74:3523—3527.
6. Fujikawa K, Hasegawa Y, Matsuzawa S, Fukunaga A, Itoh T, Kondo S. Thymus atrophy from vigorous apoptosis in p53(+/+) mice but thymus hypertrophy with no vigorous apoptosis in p53(−/−) mice after irradiation. Int J Radiat Biol (Submitted).
7. Yamamoto O, Seyama T, Jo T, Terato H, Saito T, Kinomura A. Oral administration of tritiated water (HTO) in mice. II: tumour development. Int J Radiat Biol 1995;68:47—54.
8. Yamamoto O, Seyama T, Itoh H, Fujimoto N. Oral administration of tritiated water (HTO) in mice. III: low dose-rate irradiation and threshold dose-rate for radiation risk. Int J Radiat Biol 1998;73:535—541.
9. Cohen SM, Ellwein LB. Cell proliferation in carcinogenesis. Science 1990;249:1007—1011.
10. Kondo S. Finsen Medal Lecture: Tissue-repair error model for radiation carcinogenesis. Proceedings of the 12th International Congress of Photobiology, Milano, OEMF, 1998;11—15.
11. Kondo S. Apoptotic repair of genotoxic tissue damage and the role of p53 gene. Mutation Res 1998;402:311—319.
12. Lowe SW, Bodis S, McClatchey A, Remington L, Ruley HE, Fisher DE, Housman DE, Jack T. p53 status and the efficacy of cancer therapy in vivo. Science 1994;266:807—810.
13. Kemp CJ, Wheldon T, Balmain A. p53-deficient mice are extremely susceptible to radiation-

induced tumorigenesis. Nat Genet 1994;8:66—69.

14. Cunto FD, Topley G, Calautti E, Hsiao J, Ong L, Seth PK, Dotto GP. Inhibitory function of p21$^{Cip1/WAF1}$ in differentiation of primary mouse keratinocytes independent of cell cycle control. Science 1998;280:1069—1072.

Dose-rate effect on radon-induced lung carcinogenesis

Georges Monchaux and Jean-Paul Morlier

CEA-Département de Radiobiologie et Radiopathologie, Laboratoire de Cancérologie Expérimentale, Fontenay aux Roses, France

Abstract. Experimental animal studies in addition to epidemiological studies were used to investigate the effects of exposure, exposure rate, and other factors in predicting risks resulting from human exposures to radiation. The advantage of animal data is that animal experiments are generally conducted under carefully controlled conditions and that exposure along with exposure rate can be estimated more accurately. A trend towards increasing tumour risk with decreased exposure rate was observed in rats exposed at cumulative exposures varying from about 0.72 J h m^{-3} (200 WLM) up to 10.8 J h m^{-3} (3,000 WLM), and high exposure rates varying from 0.09 J h m^{-3} (25 WLM per week) to 1.8 J m^{-3} (500 WLM per week). By contrast, the results obtained at low cumulative exposure (comparable to domestic indoor exposures) showed no evidence of an inverse exposure-rate effect.

A new series of experiments was carried out to investigate the influence of exposure rate on lung cancer induction in rats at relatively low cumulative exposures of 0.36 J h m^{-3} (100 WLM), and at a potential alpha energy concentration (PAEC) varying from 0.27 mJ m^{-3} (13 WL) to 3.15 mJ m^{-3} (150 WL). The preliminary results indicate that at relatively low cumulative exposures (comparable to lifetime exposures in high-radon houses or current underground mining exposures), the risk of lung cancer in rats decreases with decreasing PAEC, i.e., exposure rates. These data suggest that the induction of lung cancer results from a complex interplay between cumulative exposure and exposure-rate, with an optimal combination of these (two) parameters.

Keywords: cumulative exposure, exposure-rate, lung cancer, radon, radon progeny, rat.

Introduction

Epidemiological studies in uranium miners and other underground miners showed an association between an excess risk of lung cancer and exposure to radon and its progeny [1,2], but the evidence of an excess risk of lung cancer from residential radon indoor exposure is less conclusive [3]. Animal studies were carried out in addition to epidemiological studies in order to investigate the effects of exposure, exposure rate, and other factors in predicting risks resulting from human exposures (both at home and in the workplace). The advantage of animal data is that animal experiments are generally conducted under carefully controlled conditions and that exposure (and exposure-rate) can be estimated more accurately. Radon animal data obtained primarily from adult rats, was provided mainly by the Pacific Northwest Laboratory (PNNL, formerly

─────────────────────────

Address for correspondence: Dr Georges Monchaux, CEA-Département de Radiobiologie et Radio-pathologie, Laboratoire de Cancérologie Expérimentale, BP 6, F-92265 Fontenay aux Roses Cedex, France. Tel.: +33-1-46-54-70-48. Fax: +33-1-46-54-88-86. E-mail: monchaux@dsvidf.cea.fr

PNL) in USA and CEA-COGEMA in France [4]. It has been shown that the risk of lung cancer increased with increasing cumulative exposures. An excess risk of lung cancer was observed in rats at cumulative exposures as low as 0.09 J h m^{-3} (25 WLM) performed at a relatively high potential alpha energy concentration (PAEC) of 2.1 mJ m^{-3} (100 WL) [5]. A dose-effect relationship was established for cumulative exposures varying from 0.09 J h m^{-3} (25 WLM) to 10.8 J h m^{-3} (3,000 WLM), values of which were very similar for medium and high cumulative exposures observed in uranium miners [6].

In the Pacific Northwest Laboratory experiments in the USA, a trend towards an increasing tumour risk with decreased exposure-rate (also called inverse exposure-rate effect) has been reported in Wistar rats exposed at 2.1 mJ m^{-3} (100 WL) and 21 mJ m^{-3} (1,000 WL), and cumulative exposures varying from 2.3 J h m^{-3} (640 WLM) up to 18.4 J h m^{-3} (5,120 WLM) [7]. A similar trend towards increasing tumour risk with decreased exposure rate was observed in our studies [6] in Sprague-Dawley rats exposed to cumulative exposures varying from about 0.72 J h m^{-3} (200 WLM) up to 10.8 J h m^{-3} (3,000 WLM) and high exposure rates varying from 0.09 J h m^{-3} (25 WLM per week) to 1.8 J m^{-3} (500 WLM per week).

By contrast, the results obtained at low cumulative exposures, comparable to domestic indoor exposures, showed no evidence of an inverse exposure-rate effect [8]. Chronic radon exposure at 0.09 J h m^{-3} (25 WLM), protracted over an 18 months period at a PAEC of 0.042 mJ m^{-3} (2 WL), resulted in fewer cases of lung carcinoma in rats than a similar cumulative exposure protracted over 4 to 6 months at a PAEC of 2.1 mJ m^{-3} (100 WL). Moreover, the lung cancer incidence in rats exposed at low exposure rate (0.60%) was insignificantly lower than that in control animals (0.63%) [8].

Materials and Methods

Under the Fourth CEC Research and Development Framework Programme, a new series of experiments was carried out to specifically investigate the influence of exposure-rate on lung cancer induction in rats at relatively low cumulative exposures (comparable to lifetime exposures in high-radon houses or current underground mining exposures (0.36 J h m^{-3}, 100 WLM). The animal experiments were conducted concomitantly both at CEA (France) and AEA-Technology, Plc (Harwell, UK). Where possible, the experimental conditions used at the two laboratories were similar, for example both groups used rats of the same strain, sex, and age. In addition, the metrology of the radon exposure atmospheres and the reporting of pathology were standardised between the two groups. The principal difference between the exposure conditions was that exposures were conducted during the working day at CEA and continuously (24 h/day) at Harwell. The present paper reports the preliminary results of the experiments conducted at CEA.

Radon exposure

Exposures were designed to investigate the role of PAEC and protraction of exposure which have been demonstrated to be the main important parameters for lung cancer induction in experimental animals. All the CEA animal exposures were performed at the CEA-University of Limoges radon-inhalation facility located in Razès (France). Radon gas emanation from uranium ore was introduced into the 10 m^3 stainless steel chambers through a dilution system and the radon progeny were attached to the ambient aerosol (natural aerosol). The duration of exposure sessions was 6 h. Exposures were conducted under static conditions, without air renewal in the chambers. During the exposures, monitoring of the PAEC, equilibrium factor F, unattached fraction f_p, radon progeny concentrations and environmental conditions were performed using recognised methods agreed between AEA and CEA in previous metrology inter-comparison exercises [9]. Inhalation parameters of the different exposure groups are summarised in Table 1.

In these studies, experiments were performed at a cumulative exposure of 360 mJ h m^{-3} (100 WLM), and PAEC varying from 0.22 mJ m^{-3} (12–13 WL) to 3.15 mJ m^{-3} (150 WL). Group 0 (RnCt) was an unexposed control group. Group 1 (RnPC) was used as a positive control group and was exposed to radon and progeny at a cumulative exposure of about 360 mJ h m^{-3} (100 WLM) and high PAEC of 3.15 mJ m^{-3} (150 WL) which was expected to induce a lung cancer incidence of about 10%. Group 2 (RnFr) was exposed to a similar cumulative exposure of 360 mJ h m^{-3} (100 WLM) and high PAEC as Group 1, but the exposure of this group was protracted over a 3 month period at 1 or 2 sessions per week (instead of 5 sessions per week for 4 weeks as with Group 1). Group 3 (RnD3) was exposed to a similar cumulative radon exposure of 360 mJ h m^{-3}

Table 1. Distribution of rats and characteristics of exposure to radon/radon progeny within the different experimental groups.

Experimental groups	No. of rats	Age at start of exposure (months)	Cumulative exposure		PAEC		F	f_p
			mJh/m^3	WLM	mJ/m^{3U}	WL		
Gr. 0 (RnCt)[a]	120	—	≈ 0.9	≈ 0.25	≈ 0.0004	≈ 0.002	—	—
Gr. 1 (RnPC)[b]	240	3	378	105	3.91 ± 1.25	188 ± 60	0.14 ± 0.03	0.25 ± 0.04
Gr. 2 (RnFr)[c]	240	3	385	107	3.05 ± 0.95	147 ± 46	0.20 ± 0.04	0.18 ± 0.06
Gr. 3 (RnD3)[d]	240	3	361	100	1.21 ± 0.40	58.3 ± 19.4	0.09 ± 0.03	0.33 ± 0.03
Gr. 4 (RnD12)[e]	240	2.5	358	100	0.27 ± 0.01	13.0 ± 0.01	0.08 ± 0.01	0.30 ± 0.03
Gr. 5 (RnD6)[f]	211	3	151	42	0.37 ± 0.16	18.0 ± 8.0	0.14 ± 0.04	0.25 ± 0.06

[a]Group 0: untreated controls; [b]group 1: exposed to radon from 29-04-1996 to 28-05-1996; [c]group 2: exposed to radon from 11-07-1996 to 02-10-1996; [d]group 3: exposed to radon from 03-03-1997 to 03-06-1997; [e]group 4: exposed to radon from 01-12-1997 to 11-12-1998; [f]group 5: exposed to radon from 29-04-1996 to 14-10-1996.

(100 WLM), but at a lower PAEC of about 1.2 mJ m^{-3} (50 WL). Group 4 (RnD12) was exposed to a similar cumulative radon exposure of 360 mJ h m^{-3} (100 WLM), but at a PAEC of about 0.27 mJ m^{-3} (13 WL). Group 5 (RnD6) was initially scheduled to be exposed at the same cumulative exposure of 360 mJ h m^{-3} (100 WLM) as other groups, but at lower PAEC of about 0.3 mJ m^{-3} (15 WL). However, due to works for renewal and refurbishment of the radon inhalation facility, the exposure of this group was stopped at a cumulative exposure of 151 mJ h m^{-3} (42 WLM). However, this point should prove very informative, since in our experience, we had no previous data on experiments conducted at such cumulative exposures and PAEC.

Animals and histologic analysis

Exposed rats were 12 weeks of age, male, specific pathogen-free Sprague-Dawley rats (Ico: OFA SD, IFFA-CREDO, France). During exposure, they were housed in wire stainless steel cages within the inhalation chambers. Litter consisted of sawdust that was removed daily before exposure. Food (AO4 from UAR, France) and water were freely provided. After exposure, rats were kept and regularly observed until death (and euthanasied when moribund). Necropsies consisted of a complete examination of all the organs and recording any abnormalities. The lungs were carefully observed and any nodules detected by a gentle palpation. Lungs, selected organs, and organs with suspicious lesions were taken systematically for histopathological examination. Lungs were fixed in situ by intratracheal instillation of 10% neutral buffered formalin (NBF). Thoracic lymph nodes and surrounding tissues from the mediastinum, including heart, were all fixed together. If no lesions were observed, samples from liver, spleen, kidneys, and the whole brain were fixed in NBF after all the organs had been systematically weighted. Any suspicious lesion from the other organs was taken and fixed. Sagittal sections of the nasal and paranasal cavities were performed and any macroscopic lesion fixed. Tissues were fixed in NBF by immersion before processing and embedding in paraffin wax. Serial 5-μm thick sections were performed taking care to trim only sufficient tissue for histopathological diagnosis, thus making the remaining tissue from the lesion available for further studies on biological markers. Routine process consisted of haematoxylin-eosin-saffron staining. In addition, selected special histochemical stainings (including Alcian-blue for mucus detection in adenocarcinoma and/or immunohistochemical methods) were used. Proliferative preneoplastic lesions and lung tumours were classified according to the classification published in the EULEP Color Atlas [10].

Results

These studies are not as yet fully completed, however, the majority of the rats have died or were killed when moribund and then autopsied. Of the first five experimental groups, groups 1 (RnPC), 2 (RnFr), 3 (RnD3), 5 (RnD6), along with control group 0 (RnCt), all of the rats have been autopsied. By contrast, in Group 4 (RnD12), about 40% of the rats, 93 of 240, are still alive. Table 2 shows the distribution of lung tumours larger than 5 mm in diameter at macroscopic examination. In our experience, lung tumours larger than 5 mm in diameter at autopsy were found to be almost exclusively malignant tumours. In rats exposed to similar cumulative exposures and decreased PAEC, the proportion of lung tumours larger than 5 mm (at macroscopic examination) has been found to decrease from 10% in Group 1 (RnPC) to 3.33% in Group 3 (RnD3) and 1.36% in Group 4 (RnD12). However, this last group should be regarded cautiously since all the rats from this group have not yet been autopsied. On the other hand, in group 2 (RnFr), which was exposed to radon at similar cumulative exposure and similar PAEC as group 1 (RnPC) (but protracted over a 3-month period), the incidence (5.41%) of macroscopic lung tumours observed is marginally (but significantly) lower (p = 0.0896, using the Fisher's exact test) than that of Group 1 (10%). In group 5 (RnD6) exposed at lower cumulative exposure of 151 mJ h m^{-3} (42 WLM) and a lower PAEC of 0.37 mJ m^{-3} (18 WL) than other groups, 5 lung tumours larger than 5 mm at macroscopic examination (2.36%) were observed.

In these experiments, the histopathological study is still in progress. All the tumours confirmed at histopathological examination as being lung carcinomas were tumours larger than 5 mm in diameter at macroscopic examination. Until now, in group 1 (RnPC), exposed at a 378 mJ h m^{-3} (105 WLM) cumulative exposure and a high PAEC of 3.91 mJ m^{-3} (188 WL), six squamous cell carcinomas, one adenosquamous carcinoma and seven adenocarcinomas were observed. In group 2 (RnFr), exposed at a 385 mJ h m^{-3} (107 WLM) cumulative exposure and a similar PAEC of 3.06 mJ m^{-3} (147 WL) but protracted over a 3 months period, one squamous cell carcinoma, one adenosquamous carcinoma and three adenocarcinomas were observed. In group 3 (RnD3) exposed at 361 mJ h m^{-3} (100 WLM) but a lower PAEC of 1.21 mJ m^{-3} (58 WL), two papillary adenocarcinomas were observed. In group 5 (RnD6), exposed at 151 mJ h m^{-3} (42 WLM) but lower PAEC of 0.37 mJ m^{-3} (18 WL), two papillary adenocarcino-

Table 2. Distribution of macroscopic lung tumours with a diameter larger than 5 mm observed at autopsy in rats within the different experimental groups.

Experimental groups	No. of rats with lung tumours $\varnothing \geqslant 5\,mm$	No. of rats with single lung tumours	No. of rats with multiple lung tumours	Total no. of tumours $\varnothing \geqslant 5\,mm$	Proportion (%) of tumours $\varnothing \geqslant 5\,mm$
Group 0 (RnCt)[a]	0/120	0	0	0	0
Group 1 (RnPC)[b]	22/240	22	2	24	10.0
Group 2 (RnFr)[c]	13/240	13	0	13	5.41
Group 3 (RnD3)[d]	8/240	8	0	8	3.33
Group 4 (RnD12)[e]	2/147	2	0	1	1.36
Group 5 (RnD6)[f]	5/211	5	0	5	2.36

mas were also observed. It should be pointed out that squamous cell carcinomas were observed only in rats exposed at a high exposure rate.

A full statistical analysis of the survival and tumour incidence of this study will not be possible until all the animals have been analysed.

Discussion

These studies are not yet fully completed and the histopathology study is still in progress. Full statistical analysis of all animals is required before full conclusions can be drawn. However, on the basis of autopsy (macroscopic) findings and of preliminary histopathological results, the results of this study could be compared with those of an historical control group of 785 rats and with those of previous experiments in rats exposed at various cumulative exposures and exposure-rates.

The preliminary results of these studies indicate that at relatively low cumulative exposures of 0.36 J h m^{-3} (100 WLM) (comparable to lifetime exposures in high-radon houses or current underground mining exposures) the risk of lung cancer in rats decreases with PAEC, i.e., exposure-rate. They confirm the results obtained at lower cumulative exposure showing that for the same cumulative exposure of 0.09 J h m^{-3} (25 WLM), the relative risk (RR) decreases from 4.45 in rats exposed at 3.15 mJ m^{-3} (150 WL) to 3.48 in rats exposed at 2.1 mJ m^{-3} (100 WL) and to 0.94 in rats exposed at 0.042 mJ m^{-3} (2 WL). These preliminary results also indicate that the risk of lung tumour induction for rats is at a maximum for cumulative exposures ranging from 0.09 J h m^{-3} (25 WLM) up to 360 mJ h m^{-3} (100 WLM) and a PAEC ranging from 1.05 mJ m^{-3} (50 WL) up to 3.15 mJ m^{-3} (150 WL), i.e., exposure rates ranging from 18 mJ h m^{-3} per week (5 WLM per week) and 90 mJ h m^{-3} per week (25 WLM per week). These data suggest that the induction of lung cancer results from a complex interplay between cumulative exposure and exposure-rate, with an optimal combination of these (two) parameters.

The significance of exposure rates in assessing the hazards of domestic radon exposure was addressed on biophysical grounds by Brenner [11], who concluded that, when cumulative exposures are sufficiently low that multiple traversals of target cells by α particles are rare (as in the case of typical domestic radon exposures), all exposure-rate enhancement effects disappear. The results of recent experiments conducted by Miller et al. using a microbeam source [12], showed that traversal of cell nuclei by a single α-particle induced significantly lower oncogenic transformation in the C3H10T1/2 mouse fibroblast system than in a Poisson-distributed mean of one α-particle; thus suggesting that cells traversed by multiple α-particles contribute most of the risk. In this respect (based on dose-rate effect considerations) extrapolation of lower exposure-rate miner data to residential exposures (where no target cell is traversed by more than a single α-particle) may overestimate risks associated with typical residential exposures and exposure-rates. Our recent data in rats appears to follow this same trend and to support the hypothesis that, at low doses, the risk of lung cancer is governed by the rate at which the dose is delivered, and not by the total cumulative dose alone. Likewise, recent data from R. Mitchell et al. [13], following chronic exposures to high concentrations of natural uranium ore dust alone, also indicate that malignant lung tumour risks are not directly proportional to dose, but are directly proportional to dose-rate.

These data are also consistent with that of underground miners [14] showing an inverse dose-rate effect at high cumulative exposures, but a diminution of this effect at cumulative exposures lower than 0.18 J h m^{-3} (50 WLM). They support both the reality of an inverse dose-rate effect at high cumulative exposure, as well as its diminution or disappearance at low cumulative exposures.

Acknowledgements

This work was supported in part by Grant FI4P-CT95-0025 (Commission of the European Communities) and COGEMA (PIC D11).

References

1. Lubin JH, Boice JD Jr, Edling C, Hornung RW, Howe G, Kunz E, Kusiak RA, Morrison HI, Radford EP, Samet JM, Tirmarche M, Woodward A, Xiang YS, Pierce DA. Radon and Lung Cancer Risk: a Joint Analysis of 11 Underground Miners Studies. US Department of Health and Human Services, Public Health Service, Bethesda, Maryland: NIH Publication No. 94-3644, 1994.
2. Lubin JH, Boice JD Jr, Edling C, Hornung RW, Howe G, Kunz E, Kusiak RA, Morrison HI, Radford EP, Samet JM, Tirmarche M, Woodward A, Xiang YS, Pierce DA. Lung cancer in radon-exposed miners and estimation of risk from indoor radon exposure. J Natl Cancer Inst 1995;87:817–827.
3. Lubin JH, Boice JD Jr. Lung cancer risk from residential radon: meta-analysis of eight epidemiological studies. J Natl Cancer Inst 1997;89:49–57.
4. Cross FT, Monchaux G. Risk assessment of radon health effects from experimental animal studies. A joint review of PNL (USA) and CEA-COGEMA (France) data. In: Doi M, Inaba J (eds) Indoor Radon Exposure and its Health Consequences - Quest for the True story of Environmental Radon and Lung Cancer. Tokyo, Japan: Kodansha Scientific, Co. Ltd., 1999;85–105.
5. Chameaud J, Masse R, Lafuma J. Influence of radon daughter exposure at low doses on the occurrence of lung cancers in rats. Radiat Protect Dosim 1984;7:385–388.
6. Monchaux G, Morlier JP, Morin M, Chameaud J, Lafuma J, Masse R. Carcinogenic and co-carcinogenic effects of radon and radon daughters in rats. Environ Health Perspect 1994;102:64–73.
7. Gilbert ES, Cross FT, Dagle GE. Analysis of lung tumor risks in rats exposed to radon. Radiat Res 1996;145:350–360.
8. Morlier JP, Morin M, Monchaux G, Pineau JF, Chameaud J, Lafuma J, Masse R. Lung cancer incidence after exposure of rats to low doses of radon: influence of dose rate. Radiat Protect Dosim 1994;56:93–97.
9. Strong JC, Morlier JP, Monchaux G, Barstra RW, Groen JS, Baker ST. Intercomparison of measurement techniques used in radon exposure facilities for animals in Europe. Appl Radiat Isot 1996;47:355–359.
10. Hahn FF, Boorman GA. Neoplasia and preneoplasia of the lung. In: Bannasch P, Gössner W (eds) Pathology of Neoplasia and Preneoplasia in Rodents. New York: EULEP Color Atlas,

154

Volume 2, Schattauer, Stuttgart, 1997;29–42.

11. Brenner DJ. The significance of dose rate in assessing the hazards of domestic radon exposure. Health Phys 1994;67:76–79.

12. Miller RC, Randers-Pehrson G, Geard CR, Hall EJ, Brenner DJ. The oncogenic transforming potential of the passage of single α-particles through mammalian cell nuclei. Proc Natl Acad Sci USA 1999;96:19–22.

13. Mitchell RE, Jackson JS, Heinmiller B. Inhaled uranium ore dust and lung cancer risk in rats. Health Phys 1999;76:145–155.

14. Lubin JH, Boice JD Jr, Edling C, Hornung RW, Howe G, Kunz E, Kusiak RA, Morrison HI, Radford EP, Samet JM, Tirmarche M, Woodward A, Xiang YS, Pierce DA. Radon-exposed underground miners and inverse dose-rate (protraction enhancement) effects. Health Phys 1995;69:494–500.

Threshold dose in radiation carcinogenesis

Hiroshi Tanooka

National Cancer Center Research Institute, Tsukiji, Chuo-ku, Tokyo; and Central Research Institute of Electric Power Industry, Komae, Tokyo, Japan

Abstract. Arguments concerning estimation of cancer risk of ionizing radiation are often confused by ignoring the conditions of radiation exposure, especially dose-rate. To clarify the problem, a brief review of the dose-response relationships of cancer induction for various radiation exposure conditions was presented. A threshold dose, or threshold dose-rate for cancer appears under continuous exposure conditions.

Keywords: cancer, continuous exposure, dose-response, ionizing radiation.

Introduction

The question of whether the dose-response relationship in radiation carcinogenesis is linear or threshold-type is often argued. However, the question itself is not the appropriate question. What should be asked is under what conditions the dose-response approaches linearity or the threshold-type. The target theory implies that a living cell is regarded as a physical target with a certain cross-section for interaction with radiation. However, the target theory does not explain the variation in the biological response of the hit target-cell itself by modification such as DNA repair, apoptosis, and interaction with surrounding cells in the tissue. Such biological responses are thought to be dependent on dose, or the dose-rate, of radiation and to determine the final carcinogenic effects in the whole-body system. The importance of the whole-body system with regard to the dose-response in radiation carcinogenesis has been recognized [1,2]. Figure 1 illustrates the variation of dose-response relationships for cancer induction depending upon radiation exposure conditions. Actually, the threshold-type dose-response has been observed for induction of mouse tumors (with repeated radiation as an extreme case). The threshold dose-response had been previously recognized in the malformation of mice irradiated in utero during organogenesis [3], which was later proved to be dependent on the function of the *p53* gene [4].

Here I shall attempt to explain how the dose-response for cancer induction depends upon whether radiation is given to the whole body or to a part of the body, in an acute or protracted manner, or even extended to the life time, and

Address for correspondence: Hiroshi Tanooka, Genetics Division, National Cancer Center Research Institute, 511 Tsukiji, Chuo-ku, Tokyo 104-0045, Japan. Tel.: +81-3-3542-2511 (ext. 4420). Fax: +81-3-3541-2685. E-mail: htanooka@ncc.go.jp

156

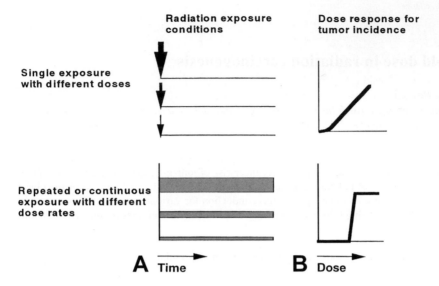

Radiation exposure conditions

Single exposure with different doses

Repeated or continuous exposure with different dose rates

A Time

Dose response for tumor incidence

B Dose

Fig. 1. Schematic illustration of time course after various radiation exposure conditions **(A)** and cancer incidence with regard to total dose given **(B)**.

propose that the dose-response in radiation carcinogenesis should be discussed at each level separately.

Cancer induction under various radiation-exposure conditions

Acute whole-body exposure with single dose

Well-known human cases are the A-bomb survivors, where leukemia is a major cancer risk. Its dose-response fits a linear-quadratic model; however, below 0.2 Gy no increase of leukemia is recognized [5] and this no-increase region is more evident [6] in Nagasaki cases [7], where the γ-ray component is predominant. Early experimental data by Upton et al. [8] showed no apparent threshold for the dose-response of the leukemia induction in mice which received acute whole-body X-irradiation.

Continuous or repeated whole-body exposure with multiple doses

The carcinogenic effect of different dose-rates of radiation has been observed strictly with a fixed total dose given over a relatively short period of time. The leukemia incidence is decreased by lowering the dose-rate for low-LET radiation, as seen in early experiments with mice [8,9]. However, this dose-rate effect is smaller for induction of solid tumors [10]. With neutrons, this decrease is absent [8]; an indication of the irrepairability caused by high-LET radiation damage. However, the lowering of the dose-rate or fractionation of the total dose necessarily involves prolongation of the exposure time and, more importantly, the process of repeated irradiation. These repeated treatments are effective in providing a higher yield of cancer, as seen in the induction of the mouse thymic lymphoma [11]. The apparent inverse dose-rate effect is seen in the transformation of cultured mouse cells in vitro with neutrons [12]. It has been known that the error-prone repair mechanism (or SOS repair) is induced by repeating the irradiation. In the whole-body system, this repeated irradiation increases the chance of tissue-misrepair or wound-healing error [6]. Therefore, the dose-response curve becomes more complex due to a higher error-free repair efficiency at low doses and a higher chance of error by the repeat at high doses, thus approaching the threshold-type. Adaptive response [13] was recognized in early observation (at the whole-body level) as acquired radiation resistance [14]. It may influence the shape of the dose-response curve.

Lifetime whole-body exposure with low doses

This is an extreme case of protracted exposure. The total accumulated dose of radiation becomes very high during the lifetime of experimental animals and humans; however, the carcinogenic effect is very low compared with that expected from short-period exposure with the same total dose. Error-free repair, adaptation, and apoptotic elimination of injured cells may be operating more efficiently at a very low dose-rate. Very few experimental data are available for this category, especially concerning the relation between cancer incidence and the total dose given. This dose-response relation is important in assessing the cancer risk of humans living in an elevated natural radiation background. Epidemiological studies are now being conducted in such areas as Yangjiang, China with a radiation level approximately 3-fold higher than that of the control area [15] and Kerala, India with a 7- to 10-fold higher level [16], where no indication of the increase of cancer risk has been recognized. Internally deposited radionuclides may be included here, however, because exposure is limited to the target organ it is better for it to be included in the category of partial-body exposure.

Acute partial-body exposure with single dose

Partial-body exposure provides a tissue with an environment in which injured cells are surrounded by uninjured cells. This circumstance creates interaction between these cells, which influences the dose-response of the final cancer incidence. A relatively large number of experimental data are available for this category. For example, the tumor incidence in rat skin by single doses of β-rays increases with dose up to a peak at 30 Gy (with no apparent threshold) [17], whereas the dose-response for lung cancer incidence by a single exposure of the chest (of mice) to X-rays shows no increase of cancer up to 2 Gy, and starts to rise with higher doses in a threshold manner [18].

Continuous or repeated partial-body exposure with multiple doses

A higher repair efficiency at a low dose and at a low dose-rate (and the higher chance of error by the repeat of exposure) are more enhanced in the partial-body exposure than in the whole-body exposure. It should be noted that ionizing radiation exerts a tumor-promoting activity when repeated, and that the dose-response for tumor induction of chemical tumor promoters applied to mouse skin after application of a tumor initiator is of threshold-type [19]. A tumor initiating agent is also known to exert tumor-promoting activity when repeatedly applied.

Lifetime partial-body exposure

Lifetime exposure yields an extreme case of protracted or repeated exposures. Mice which do not develop skin cancer with single doses of β-rays develop skin and bone tumors with 100% efficiency by repeating a dose of 1 Gy (or more) 3 times weekly. However, with 0.5 Gy (total dose: 150 Gy in 2 years) no tumors develop over a lifetime, showing a threshold type dose-response [20—24]. It is indicated that the carcinogenic effect of 0.5 Gy per exposure was completely eliminated during 2—3 days using this system.

Internally deposited radionuclides with a long half-life are also included in this category, since they irradiate the target organs continuously. Tritiated water administered to mice induces lymphomas with a threshold-type dose response [25]. In radium painters, the dose-response for bone-tumor incidence shows a wide dose range of the zero level and a sharp rise at an accumulated dose of 10 Gy [26]. High-LET radiation has been thought to produce irreparable damage, and for this reason its carcinogenic effect is expected to have no dose-rate dependency. In this regard, indoor radon has been considered a major source of lung cancer in a natural radiation environment. However, Morlier et al. [27] demonstrated that the lung cancer incidence for the same total doses of radon administered to rats diminished to the control level when the radon concentration was reduced to a low dose-rate range, thus indicating the presence of a dose-rate effect even for high-LET radiation. In this regard, the RBE value of high-LET radiation for cancer induction at a low dose-rate should be revised.

The magnitude of the threshold dose for cancers varies depending upon target organs, and the molecular mechanism of the threshold response involves DNA repair and cellular apoptosis [28]. Furthermore, adaptive response and immunological response of the whole body should be involved. This situation holds true not only for ionizing radiation but also for other types of environmental carcinogens.

Conclusion

The cancer risk of ionizing radiation should be discussed separately for different exposure conditions with various dose-response relations. The threshold dose-response is characteristic of continuous exposure to low dose-rate radiation.

Acknowledgements

I wish to thank Dr S. Kondo, Atomic Energy Research Institute, Kinki University; Dr T. Yamada, Central Research Institute of Electric Power Industry, and Dr R.J.M. Fry, Oak Ridge National Laboratory for valuable suggestions.

References

1. Upton AC, Albert RE, Burns FJ, Shore RE (eds) Radiation Carcinogenesis. New York: Elsevier Science B.V., 1986.
2. Yokoro K, Fry RJM, Kondo S, Sado T, Tanooka H. Radiation carcinogenesis in the whole body system. Radiat Res 1991;32(Suppl 2).
3. Nomura T. High sensitivity of fertilized eggs to radiation and chemicals in mice: comparison with that of germ cells and embryos at organogenesis. Congen Anomaly 1984;24:329—337.
4. Norimura T, Nomoto S, Katsuki M, Gondo Y, Kondo S. p53-Dependent apoptosis suppresses radiation-induced teratogenesis. Nature Med 1996;2:577—580.
5. Shimizu Y, Kato H, Schull WJ. Studies of the mortality of A-bomb survivors. Report mortality, 1950—1985: Part 2. Cancer mortality based on the recently revised doses (DS86). Radiat Res 1990;121:120—141.
6. Kondo S. Health Effects of Low-Level Radiation. Osaka: Kinki University Press, and Madison: Medical Physics Publishing, 1993.
7. Ichimaru M, Tomonaga M, Amenomori T, Matsuo T. Atomic bomb and leukemia. Radiat Res 1991;32(Suppl 2):14—19.
8. Upton A, Randolph ML, Conklin JW. Late effects of fast neutrons and γ-rays in mice as influenced by the dose rate of irradiation: induction of neoplasm. Radiat Res 1970;41:467—491.
9. Mole RH. Patterns of response to whole-body irradiation: the effect of dose and exposure time on duration of life and tumour production. Br J Radiol 1959;32:497—501.
10. Ullrich RL, Storer JB. Influence of γ-radiation on the development of neoplastic disease in mice. III: dose-rate effects. Radiat Res 1979;80:325—342.
11. Kaplan HS. Observations on radiation-induced lymphoid tumors of mice. Cancer Res 1947;7: 141—147.
12. Hill CK, Carnes BA, Han A, Elkind MM. Neoplastic transformation is enhanced by multiple low doses of fission-spectrum neutrons. Radiat Res 1985;102:404—410.
13. Olivieri G, Bodycote J, Wolff S. Adaptive response of human lymphocytes to low concentrations of radioactive thymidine. Science 1984;223:594—597.
14. Quastler H, Bensted JPM, Chir B, Lamerton LF, Simpson SM. Adaptation to continuous irradiation: observations on the rat intestine. Br J Radiol 1959;32:501—512.
15. Chen DQ, Wei LX. Chromosome aberrations, cancer mortality and hormetic phenomena among inhabitants in areas of high background radiation in China. Radiat Res 1991;32(Suppl 2):46—53.
16. Nair MK, Nambi KSV, Amma NS, Gangdharan P, Jayalekshmi P, Jayadevan S, Chrian V, Reghuram KN. Population study in the high natural background radiation area in Kerala, India. Radiat Res 1999;152(Suppl):S145—S148.
17. Albert RE, Neuman W, Altshuler B. The dose-response relationships of β-ray induced skin tumors in the rat. Radiat Res 1961;15:410—430.
18. Ullrich RL, Jernigan MC, Adams LM. Induction of lung tumors in RFM mice after localized exposures to X-rays and neutrons. Radiat Res 1979;80:464—473.

19. Hecker E, Rippmann F. Outline of a descriptive general theory of environmental chemical cancerogenesis-experimental threshold doses for tumor promoters. In: Kappas A (ed) Mechanisms of Environmental Mutagenesis Carcinogenesis. New York: Plenum, 1990;167—173.

20. Ootsuyama A, Tanooka H. Threshold-like dose of local beta irradiation repeated throughout the life span of mice for induction of skin and bone tumors. Radiat Res 1991;125:98—101.

21. Ootsuyama A, Tanooka H. Zero tumor incidence in mice after repeated lifetime exposures to 0.5 Gy of β-radiation. Radiat Res 1993;134:244—246.

22. Tanooka H, Ootsuyama A. Non-linear threshold dose response of murine tumorigenesis by repeated β-irradiation and p53 mutations involved. In: Hagen U, Harder D, Jung H, Streffer C (eds) Radiation Research 1895—1995. Würzburg: 10th international congress of radiation research, 1995;693—696.

23. Tanooka H, Ootsuyama A, Sasaki H. Homologous recombination between p53 and its pseudogene in a radiation-induced mouse tumor. Cancer Res 1998;58:5649—5651.

24. Tanooka H. Biological effects of low doses of radiation. In: Baumstark-Khan C, Kozubek S, Horneck G (eds) Fundamentals for the Assessment of Risks from Environmental Radiation. Dordrecht, Boston, London: Kluwer Academic Publishers, 1999;471—478.

25. Yamamoto O, Seyama T, Itoh H, Fujimoto N. Oral administration of tritiated water in mouse. III: low dose-rate irradiation and threshold dose-rate for radiation risk. Int J Radiat Biol 1998; 73:535—541.

26. Rowland RE. Dose response relationships for female radium dial workers: a new look. In: van Kaick G, Karaoglou A, Kellerer AM (eds) Health Effects of Internally Deposited Radionuclides: Emphasis on Radium and Thorium. Singapore, New Jersey, London, Hong Kong: World Scientific, 1994;181—191.

27. Morlier JP, Morin M, Monchaux G, Pineau G, Chameaud JF, Lafuma J, Masse R. Lung cancer incidence after exposure of rats to low doses of radon: influence of dose rate. Radiat Protect Dosimet 1994;56:93—97.

28. Kondo S. Evidence that there are threshold effects in risk of radiation. J Nucl Sci Tech 1999;36: 1—9.

29. Kondo S. Threshold effects arising from concerted DNA repair and apoptosis. Radiat Res (In press).

Threshold dose and dose-rate for thymic lymphoma induction and life shortening in mice administered tritiated drinking water

Osamu Yamamoto[1] and Toshio Seyama[2]

[1] Hiroshima International University, Hiroshima; and [2] Yasuda Women's University, Hiroshima, Japan

Abstract. Female (C57BL/6N and C3H/He) F_1 mice were maintained for their entire life span (or for different durations) on drinking water containing various levels of tritiated water (HTO), the dose/dose-rate dependency of tumor induction and life shortening was examined. The dose and dose-rate response for thymic lymphoma induction was threshold type. Incidence of the lymphoma declined to zero level by decreasing the total dose or dose-rate below 5 Gy or 12 mGy per day respectively. The threshold dose and threshold dose-rate for life shortening were also found at 1 Gy and 2 mGy per day.

Keywords: dose (dose-rate) dependency, HTO, life span, tumor induction.

Background

The linear nonthreshold dose-response model is now widely accepted as a paradigm in radiation biology, although the dose-response curve could not be practically determined at low dose levels. Especially no data concerning very low dose rates are available. Studies on mice given tritiated water as drinking water for the entire life span make it possible to study the dose-effect relationship in the very low dose range.

This paper summarizes the results concerning the existence of a threshold dose and dose-rate for induction of thymic lymphoma and life shortening of mice given tritiated drinking water at various concentrations, the experimental details of which were described previously [1–3].

Materials and Methods

Ten-week-old female (C57BL/6N and C3H/He, Charles River Japan) F_1 mice were selected and maintained for their entire life span on drinking water containing various levels of HTO (Amarsham). To determine organ doses, the ^3H radio-activities in blood and various organs such as the brain, liver, muscles, lungs, spleen, and kidneys were measured at regular intervals after the onset of HTO administration [2,3]. The organ dose per day can be calculated using the following equation:

Address for correspondence: Dr Osamu Yamamoto, Faculty of Health Sciences, Hiroshima International University, 555-36 Gakuendai, Kurose-cho, Kamo-gun, Hiroshima 724-0695, Japan. Tel.: +81-823-70-4581. Fax: +81-82-222-5356. E-mail: o-yama@hs.hirokoku-u.ac.jp

Organ dose per day (Gy) = specific radioactivity (Bq/g) × 5.7 keV/g (= 9.13 × 10^{13} Gy) × 60 × 60 × 24.

Finally, a complete autopsy was performed immediately upon the death of the mice, and paraffin-embedded tissue sections were stained with Hematoxylin-Eosin for the pathological analysis.

Results

Within the dose-rate range 240 to 9.6 mGy/day tumor development was the main cause of death and its incidence was found to be 70—80% as shown in Table 1. Within the range 240 mGy/day to 96 mGy/day, mice died mainly by thymic lymphoma. Incidence of the thymic lymphoma sharply decreased concomitant with an increase in other types of tumor at a dose-rate lower than 48 mGy/day. Consequently, tumor type became more diverse in the lower dose-rate range.

These changes are more clearly seen in Fig. 1. Thymic lymphoma frequency decreased as the dose rate decreased, and tumors other than thymic lymphoma increased markedly, showing a straight line in semi-log scale. It is of interest to note that the total tumor incidence remained at the same level at dose-rate ranges higher than 10 mGy/day. The level declined gradually from 70—80% to the control level (50%) by further decreases in dose-rate. The dotted straight line representing the decrease of thymic lymphoma (open circle) crosses the base line at 12 mGy/day. These results indicate clearly the existence of the threshold dose rate for thymic lymphoma.

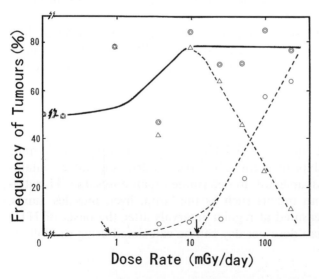

Fig. 1. Relationship of the frequency of tumors to the dose rate of ^{3}H β-irradiation. ○: Thymic lymphoma; Δ: tumors other than thymic lymphoma; ◎: total tumors. The solid arrow represents the threshold dose-rate; the dotted arrow, the tail threshold dose rate.

Table 1. Tumor development in mice at different dose-rates of HTO.

Dose-rate (mGy/day)	240	96	48	24	10	0 (A)
Cumulative dose (Gy)	38.8	34.6	19.7	11.5	5.9	0
Number of mice used	45	38	60	60	53	67
MST ± SD (day)	165 ± 36	259 ± 52	414 ± 112	481 ± 112	622 ± 121	811 ± 134
Thymic lymphoma	29 (64) [162 ± 28]	22 (58) [273 ± 51]	15 (25) [415 ± 53]	4 (7) [508 ± 202]	3 (6) [589 ± 32]	0 (0)
Nonthymic lymphoma	5 (11) [146 ± 27]	4 (11) [229 ± 24]	12 (20) [443 ± 53]	9 (15) [504 ± 32]	11 (21) [609 ± 70]	12 (18) [787 ± 129]
Reticular cell neoplasm		2 (5) [179 ± 15]	5 (8) [390 ± 67]	12 (20) [485 ± 144]	10 (19) [570 ± 150]	4 (6) [760 ± 161]
Ovarian tumor		2 (5) [201 ± 18]	4 (7) [431 ± 60]	8 (13) [511 ± 98]	11 (21) [641 ± 114]	4 (6) [868 ± 149]
Hemangiosarcoma		2 (5) [331 ± 21]				
Fibrosarcoma			2 (3) [431 ± 58]	4 (7) [467 ± 97]	6 (11) [607 ± 90]	5 (7) [868 ± 149]
Harderian gland tumor			2 (3) [423 ± 81]	2 (3) [537 ± 75]		
Lung tumor			1 (2) [464]	3 (5) [460 ± 30]	8 (15) [736 ± 84]	3 (4) [811 ± 24]
Skin tumor			1 (2) [401]			
Bladder tumor				1 (2) [580]		
Rhabdomyosarcoma				1 (2) [298]		
Mammary tumor					2 (4) [582 ± 58]	
Hepatic tumor					2 (4) [685 ± 23]	6 (9) [800 ± 151]
Adrenal tumor					1 (2) [623]	
Splenic tumor						2 (3) [827 ± 19]
Stomach tumor						1 (2) [912]
Double tumor-bearing	0 (0)	0 (0)	0 (0)	2 (3)	10 (19)	4 (6)
Tumor-carrying mice	34 (76)	32 (84)	42 (70)	42 (70)	44 (83)	33 (48)

Note: ( ) = % tumor development; [ ] = mean latent period; MST = mean survival time or mean time of death after the initial exposure; SD = standard deviation.

164

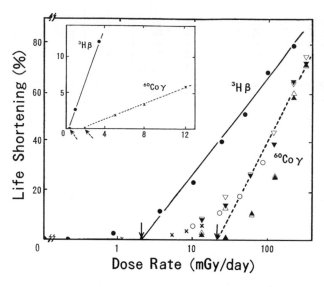

Fig. 2. Relationship of life-shortening to dose-rate of ^{3}H β-irradiation (●) in the present study with (C57BL/6N x C3H/He)F$_1$, compared with that of ^{60}Co γ-irradiation with various mouse strains: (○) for LAF1 6, 7; (▲) for A/Jax; (▼) for BALB/c; (△) for C57BL/6; (▽) for BCF$_1$, (×) for average of the above four kinds of mice (NCRP 1980) which were calculated from each MST. The solid arrow represents threshold dose-rate; the dotted arrow, tail threshold dose-rate. The two axes of the inner graph, in which the low dose-rate date were replotted to a normal scale, are the same to those of the outer graph.

Relationship between life shortening and dose-rate is shown in Fig. 2. The straight line, which can also be obtained using a semi-log scale, crossed the base line at 2 mGy/day. Thus, there also exists a threshold dose-rate for life shortening (2 mGy/day). Life shortening data reported for γ-irradiation (Lorenz et al. [4], Failla and McClement [5], Grhan et al. [6] and NCRP [7]) were plotted on the same Figure (open and closed triangles with dotted line). The dotted straight line (to the right of the solid line) was obtained at a range much higher than that for ^{3}H β-rays. The threshold dose-rates, 20 mGy/day were also found for γ-ray induced life shortening, suggesting that ^{3}H β-rays are more than ten times effective than γ-rays in terms of life shortening.

Table 2 shows results of the experiment in which the duration of HTO administration (240 mGy/day) was changed to cover a range from 90 to 10 days. When the duration was longer than 60 days, the incidence of thymic lymphoma was very high. Decreasing the length of the administration period to 30 or 10 days caused a marked decline in the incidence. In Fig. 3, incidence of thymic lymphoma and percentage of life shortening were plotted against the total accumulated dose. It is clear that the threshold doses for lymphoma induction and life shortening were 5 and 1 Gy respectively.

Table 2. Tumor developments by HTO administration for various durations at the dose-rate of 240 mGy/day.

Exposure duration (total dose)	Whole life span (39.9 Gy)	90 days (21.6 Gy)	60 days (14.4 Gy)	30 days (7.2 Gy)	10 days (2.4 Gy)
Number of mice used	45	64	62	62	64
MST, day	165	150	176	515	691
Thymic lymphoma	29 (64) [162 ± 28]	45 (70) [142 ± 25]	44 (71) [170 ± 31]	4 (6) [204 ± 20]	1 (2) [738]
Nonthymic lymphoma	5 (11) [146 ± 27]	2 (3) [151 ± 32]	2 (3) [177 ± 30]	10 (16) [493 ± 174]	8 (3) [713 ± 119]
Lung tumor		1 (2) [117]	1 (2) [179]	4 (6) [692 ± 88]	2 (3) [683 ± 41]
Fibrosarcoma			1 (2) [180]	2 (3) [553 ± 99]	8 (13) [690 ± 185]
Reticular cell neoplasm				10 (16) [516 ± 111]	6 (9) [699 ± 121]
Ovarian tumor				10 (16) [618 ± 150]	16 (25) [686 ± 168]
Liver tumor				2 (3) [754 ± 101]	4 (6) [735 ± 107]
Glanulosa cell tumor					2 (3) [628 ± 231]
Skin tumor					1 (2) [801]
Double tumor-bearing	0 (0)	0 (0)	0 (0)	2 (3)	4 (6)
Tumor-carrying mice	34 (76)	48 (74)	48 (75)	40 (65)	44 (69)

Note: ( ) = % tumor development; [ ] = mean latency; MST = mean survival time or mean time of death after the initiation of exposure; SD = standard deviation.

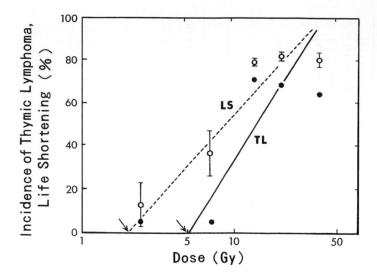

Fig. 3. Relationship of the thymic lymphoma incidence and the life shortening to the exposure duration or to the total cumulative dose at 240 mGy/day in ³H β-irradiation. ●: Thymic lymphoma; ○: life shortening.

Discussion

The linear nonthreshold model has (generally) been adopted for the risk assessment of low-dose radiation [8]. Recently, however, the validity of this model has come under question (on the basis of epidemiological studies on high background area residents). For this reason, the need for studies on radiation carcinogenesis at low doses as well as low dose-rate ranges has been emphasized [9,10]. Existence of the threshold dose or dose-rate has been discussed from the viewpoints of apoptosis [11,12]. In fact, some reported results are suggestive as to the threshold dose using small experimental animals [13,14]. In the case of thymic carcinogenesis and life shortening in F_1 mice (C57BL/6N and C3H/He), the shape and structure of the dose-response regression curve over the entire life span does not fit the linear-nonthreshold model (Figs. 1–3).

Conclusion

The present HTO-administered mouse data strongly support the existence of a threshold dose and threshold dose-rate in radiation carcinogenesis as well as in life shortening. This result will make a strong impact on radiation risk assessment.

References

1. Yamamoto O, Yokoro K, Seyama T. HTO oral administration in mice: threshold dose rate for haematopoietic death. Int J Radiat Biol 1990;57:543–549.

2. Yamamoto O, Seyama T, Terato TjoH, Saito H, Kinomura A. Oral administration of tritiated water (HTO) in mouse. II: Tumour development. Int J Radiat Biol 1995;68:47—54.

3. Yamamoto O, Seyama T, Itoh H, Fujimoto N. Oral administration of tritiated water (HTO) in mouse. III: Low dose rate irradiation and threshold dose-rate for radiation risk. Int J Radiat Biol 1998;73:535—541.

4. Lorenz E, Jacobson LO, Heston WE, Shimkin M, Eschenbrenner AB, Deringer MK, Doniger J, Schweisthal R. Effects of long-continued total body gamma irradiation on mice, guinea pigs and rabbits. III. Effects on life span, weight, blood picture, and carcinogenesis and the role of the intensity of radiation. In: Zirkle RE (ed) Biological Effects of External X and Gamma Radiation part 1. New York: McGraw-Hill, 1954;24—148.

5. Failla G, McClement P. The shortening of life by chronic whole-body irradiation. Am J Roentgenol 1957;78:946—954.

6. Grahn D, Sacher GA, Rust JH, Fry RJM. Duration of life with daily ^{60}Co gamma irradiation: report on survival and incidence of tumors. In: Argonne National Laboratory, Biological and Medical Division Annual Report ANL-7635. Lemont: Argonne National Laboratory, 1969;1—9.

7. NCRP. Report No. 64, Effects on life span. Tumorigenesis in experimental laboratory animals. In: NCRP (ed) Influence of Dose and Its Distribution in Time on Dose-Relationships for Low LET Radiation. National Council on Radiation Protection and Measurements, 1980;95—131.

8. Pierce DA, Shimizu Y, Preston DL, Vaeth M, Mabuchi K. Studies of the mortality of atomic bomb survivors. Report 12 part I. Cancer:1950—1990. Radiat Res 1996;146:1—27.

9. Abelson PH. Risk assessment of low-level exposures. Science 1994;265:1507.

10. Jovanovich JV. Radiation protection philosophy: time for changes? La Physique an Canada 1995;juillet/aout:245—265.

11. Norimura T, Nomoto S, Katsumi M, Gondo Y, Kondo S. p53 dependent apoptosis suppresses radiation-induced teratogenesis. Nature Med 1993;2:577—580.

12. Kondo S. Empirical rules for radiation-induced teratogenesis and defense mechanisms against teratogenic injury. In: Kondo S. (Author) Health. Effects of Low-Level Radiation. Madison: Medical Physics Publishing Co., 1993;73—89.

13. Ootsuyama A, Tanooka H. Zero tumor incidence in mice after repeated lifetime exposures to 0.5 Gy of beta radiation. Radiat Res 1993;134:244—246.

14. Moncheaux G, Morlier JP, Morin M, Chameaud J, Lafuma J, Masse R. Carcinogenic and co-carcinogenic effects of radon and radon daughters in rats. Environ Health Perspect 1994;102:64—73.

How dangerous is residential radon?

Klaus Becker

Radiation, Science & Health Inc., Berlin, Germany

Abstract. The question whether radon in above-ground situations represents a health hazard is important not only because of the high economical and social costs associated with the reduction of radon levels in homes, in the remediation of former uranium mining areas (e.g. in Saxony, Eastern Germany), etc., but, perhaps more importantly, because the radon controversy is becoming a test case for the validity of the LNT hypothesis, the collective dose concept, current RBE estimates, and other central issues of legislation and regulatory control regarding low radiation doses. On the one hand, official and semi-official institutions such as ICRP, NRPB, and NRC (BEIR VI) claim, based on some miners' and other epidemiological studies, that large numbers of additional lung cancers in the population are due to increased radon levels. On the other hand, various recent studies, e.g., with never-smoking women in high residential radon areas in Saxony, as well as animal and cell experiments (and theoretical models), strongly support biopositive effects, including the reduction not only of lung cancer, but also of leukemia and other types of cancer in areas with increased residential radon levels.

Keywords: cost/benefit analysis, lung cancer, radon, residential radon, risk assessment.

The paper surveys recent data with the following main results:
1. There is no international agreement regarding suggested intervention levels for residential radon.
2. Linear extrapolation from very high miner exposures to low levels in homes is not feasible because of the many confounding effects in mines.
3. Epidemiological studies indicating an increased risk of lung cancer are subject to substantial errors, in particular regarding the retrospective determination of smoking habits.
4. There is evidence for a U-shaped dose-effect relationship, with a biopositive minimum between about 200 and 1,000 Bq/m.
5. In all but a few exceptional cases, the cost/benefit ratio does not justify residential radon remediation programs.
6. These findings have obvious consequences for low dose radiation risk assessment and regulatory control, as well as for radiation protection in general and risk/benefit assessment.

Address for correspondence: Klaus Becker, Radiation, Science & Health Inc., Boothstr. 27, D-12207 Berlin, Germany. Tel.: +49-30-772-1284. Fax: +49-30-772-1284.
E-mail: prof.dr.klaus.becker@t-online.de

Introduction

Potential lung cancer risks due to the inhalation of radon daughter products (usually simply called "radon") have been the subject of wide concern in recent years, not only because of the potential impact on the well-being of people living or working in high-level radon environments, but also because of the high costs of radon remediation programs, e.g., regarding uranium mines and private homes. Recommended or mandatory intervention levels vary widely between 150 and 600 Bq/m in homes, and 600–1,000 Bq/m at the working place. Assuming an average around 250 Bq/m, this value is exceeded in a country such as Germany by 200,000 residences totalling about 800,000 people. Radon reduction program costs currently range from US$2,500 to US$25,000, with up to US$ 130,000 for a building in Austria. It is worth noting that 200–250 Bq/m, as currently discussed by the EU as a European standard, would correspond (according to ICRP) to approximately 10 mSv p.a. population dose, to be compared to 1 mSv p.a. as a limit for external radiation.

Besides the obvious economical, social, and psychological implications, the assessment of potential residential radon risk is an important test case for the validity of the linear-no-threshold (LNT) hypothesis (and the related Collective Dose concept), the RBE of high-LET radiation, the power of epidemiological studies, and other important regulatory concepts in radiation protection.

Consequently, there have been numerous conferences and publications on this subject (see, for example [1–4]) with papers describing radon concentrations in all possible enclosed spaces (not excluding ancient Egyptian tombs). However, most of them have been written by physicists measuring and/or trying to reduce radon exposures. Almost none of them seem to doubt the official paradigm that inhaled radon daughters represent a lung cancer hazard down to infinitesimal small concentrations. This point of view has recently been endorsed with estimates that about 5% of all lung cancers in England are due to residential radon, with a 40% risk increase for 400 Bq/m [5], and another report [6] attributing 15,700 to 23,600 lung cancers annually in the US to residential radon. It is the purpose of this paper to critically review the soundness of such claims.

Therapeutic radon effects?

Before an international symposium "Radon and Health" in Austria last year [7,8], some of the attending scientists from Europe, Japan, and the USA used the opportunity to visit the underground medical radon treatment facilities in Bad Gastein, where thousands of patients are treated annually for rheumatic and arthritic diseases (such as Morbus Bechterew) at a cost of about US$500 for 10 h radon inhalation at a concentration of 160,000 Bq/m. A total of approximately 75,000 patients annually undergo radon treatment by inhalation, bathes, or drinking radon-rich water in Germany and Austria. Actually, radon may be one of mankinds oldest natural remedies, dating back to ancient cultures and prehistoric times long before radon and radiation were known. In the center of the Russian uranium mining activities in Saxony (former East Germany), where presently about US$2,000 million are being spent on overground radon remediation efforts, the well-known old radon spa Bad Schlema was officially reopened last year.

It is well known that there was a period in the 1920s and 1930s in which almost every disorder was claimed to be curable with ionizing radiation, in particular radium and radon. Such transient medical fashions can survive for long periods in paramedicine (as exemplified by homeopathy and the many practices of traditional and Asian medicine, etc.), however, the beneficial effects of radon balneology now appear to be well established with several randomized double-blind studies; studies which cannot simply be explained by psychosomatic or placebo effects [7], even if the many details regarding the mechanism of such effects require further investigation.

The case of Saxony

An interesting, not yet internationally well-known area for studying residential radon effects is the area around Schneeberg in the Ore Mountains (Erzgebirge) of Southern Saxony. In 1537, the famous physician Theophrast Bombast von Hohenheim, better known as Paracelsus (who first stated "It is the dose which makes the poison") described a high incidence of a lung disease ("Bergsucht") among silver miners there. In these mines, there was a high occurrence of pitchblende, a uranium ore in which Klapproth discovered uranium more than 200 years ago, and the Curies radium 100 years ago.

This old miner's disease was identified as lung cancer 120 years ago, and in 1913 first related to the extremely high radon levels, in some cases exceeding 2 million Bq/m (or four orders of magnitude above the recommended limits in some countries [9]). In homes within this area, up to 115,000 Bq/m have been measured, and 12% of all houses exceed 15,000 Bq/m (or 100 times the US limit). Nevertheless, lung cancer remained extremely rare in the population before mass consumption of cigarettes started with the opening of Germany's first cigarette factory in Saxony in 1862.

As W. Schüttmann, the doyen of German radon lung cancer research, pointed out in a recent study [10], among the 20,000 autopsies performed at one of Saxony's largest hospitals at a time when it was already well diagnosable, the percentage of lung cancers slowly increased during the following decades. It rose from only 0.06% between 1852 and 1876 to 0.21% from 1877 to 1884. Between 1885 and 1894, this number had risen to 0.43%, and currently about one third of all exogenous cancers in Germany are attributed to smoking. WHO estimates that the worldwide average will reach 50% within a few years.

After 1945, the former Soviet Union created, with the usual total disregard for human lives and the environment, history's largest source of nuclear armament by mining about 220,000 tons of uranium, primarily in the Schneeberg/Schlema region in Saxony. These operations ceased only after the collapse of socialism in 1990. In particular during the initial "wild years" 1945–1953 (also called "Klondike in the Erzgebirge"), about 250,000 to 300,000 miners were exposed to very high radon levels, in many cases exceeding 500 WLM (which corresponds to about 5 Sv/y according to the current ICRP estimates). Probably more importantly, the miners had to survive a multitude of other severe health risks including toxic ore and dust because of dry drilling, diesel exhaust fumes, nitrous gases from blasting during the shifts, etc. Moreover, unlike the normal population (unable to afford the luxury of smoking during the starvation years after WW II) at least 80% of the miners were provided with enough benefits to indulge in heavy smoking and drinking.

As was also observed in the nearby Czech uranium mines, the above synergistic effects resulted in a definite increase in lung cancer incidence (by several thousand), even if it is impossible to distinguish between confounding and radon effects. Such miner data have later been used for a linear extrapolation down to low residential exposures. The multiplication of low concentrations with large population numbers thus resulted in the frightening estimates which can be found in ICRP recommendations and other official (and semiofficial) national and international documents. As costly remediation and construction regulations are being implemented, they are (increasingly) becoming the subject of scientific criticism. For example, beginning with German unification in 1990, about 2,000 million US$ were being spent on overground radon assessment and remediation programs. This was initially appreciated not only by a booming "radon industry" (e.g., 300 million tons of overburden have been moved and/or covered by protective layers in order to reduce radon in the ambient air), but also by the local population in an economically depressed area. However, frightening reports in the media ("Valley of Death") also seriously damaged outside investments and tourism, caused the emigration of many young and qualified people, and psychological stress for families living (in some cases already for centuries) without detrimental health effects in houses far exceeding the proposed legal limits.

Residential radon

In the years following German unification, the comprehensive cancer register of the former German Democratic Republic has been analyzed with no indication of increased female lung cancer in the high residential radon areas. With at least 90% of the women in the high-radon areas being never-smokers at this time, and the radon levels exceeding the national average by factors of 3 to 10, a substantial increase should have been expected. However, a careful investigation, recently completed for the EU ("Schneeberg Study") [11], confirmed (for the raw as well as the stratified epidemiological data) that there might be a threshold for residential radon effects on lung cancer well over 1,000 Bq/m.

In earlier studies [9], the incidence of nonsmoking female lung cancer expected from the country (averaged between 1983 and 1987) had been compared with those in the high radon districts, and approximately half the number of incidences (67 instead of 111) was observed. Moreover, despite an external gamma exposure of 1−7 mSv p.a. and a radon exposure (according to ICRP) of 10−100 mSv p.a. (sometimes more) in these areas, there is not a single case of childhood leukemia, as well as strong indications for a reduced incidence of various other types of solid cancers [12]. Despite controversies about the relative merits and power of different types of epidemiological investigations (it has been repeatedly explained by epidemiologists that this is an unreliable tool for risk factors below 2 to 3) there is increasing evidence that some case control studies, which served as the basis for current recommendations and regulations, are highly questionable. There have, for example, been studies in the US supporting Cohen's much disputed findings [13].

Such developments raise a number of interesting questions. For example, should we really trust the hypothesis that detrimental effects in miners can be extrapolated linearly down to zero levels? Even BEIR VI does not exclude the possibility of a threshold value, there are reasonable mechanistic models consistent with a U-shaped dose-response relationship for radon [14], and a prominent radiation protection expert recently concluded [6] that "epidemiological evidence to support (EPA) conclusions is either absent or not convincing. A more reasonable conclusion is that lung cancer risk is insignificant for radon concentrations below 400 Bq/m. Radon does not pose a threat to the public health in the domestic environment." This confirms a suspicion which was already expressed over a decade ago, that "with radon an artificial disease has been created by the multiplication of a very small risk with large populations, in order to obtain frightening numbers" [15].

There is much research data, to directly or indirectly support such conclusions, e.g.,
1) the relative risk of lung cancer for external low-LET exposures decreases, contrary to the LNT hypothesis, before reaching a threshold around 2 Gy [16];
2) experimental animal studies demonstrate an RBE for lung cancer induction by α-radiation of 2 instead of 20 as assumed by ICRP [17];
3) further experimental evidence for a definitely non-linear radon effect, amounting to an overestimation of residential radon risks, was recently provided in single alpha particle exposures of mammalian cells [18]; and
4) regarding incorporated alpha emitters such as Ra and Pu in humans and animals, there is substantial evidence supporting no detectable effect up to at least 2−4 Gy.

Discussion and Conclusions

If a clearer, but quite different in terms of currently prevailing "official" assumption, picture is emerging from the pieces of the residential radon puzzle, then this will imply consequences for the assessment of low-dose effects in general (including the collective dose paradigm, RBE, etc.), and could have far-reaching consequences for the future regarding, e.g., the cost/benefit analysis of nuclear waste and remediation programs, the public acceptance of nuclear power, radiation uses in medicine and research, etc. It could affect basic administrative and regulatory procedures, as well as stimulate research on epidemiology in high natural radiation areas, adaptive response, DNA repair mechanisms, etc.

Naturally, the results of epidemiological studies, not only in China, Canada, Finland, etc. (which, like those in Saxony, show no bionegative or even biopositive effects for radon levels up to about 1,000 Bq/m), but also those of other residential radon studies in Sweden, Germany, and Southwest England (which appear to indicate a slight lung cancer risk) deserve serious consideration. It is evident that almost all such studies are subject to large uncertainties: the statistical power of the relatively few cases is low in the high radon categories, and there remain extensive uncertainties in radon dosimetry under actual field conditions. For example, the team responsible for a US$10 million study in Germany stated in a recent publication [19] that "radon was not considered a risk factor, because it is a weak risk factor."

More importantly, the retrospective evaluation of smoking habits is subject to large uncertainties. It has been shown that cigarette addicts (perhaps even more than other addictive drug users) notoriously underestimate their consumption, in particular after lung cancer has been diagnosed. It was also pointed out that underestimation of only one cigarette per day would already invalidate some of the well-known case control studies. Consequently, with very costly residential radon remediation programs in the USA and in Europe already in progress or under consideration, there emerges an important question: could and should such funds not be better used for the reduction of clearly established public health hazards in the world's affluent, and even more so in the less affluent, countries?

The current residential radon situation may be summarized as follows:

1. The regulatory situation is inconsistent, with suggested intervention levels fluctuating between countries (by large factors), and ICRP recommending a radon limit for the population which is a factor of 10 larger than that for external γ-radiation.

2. The underlying linear extrapolation from high miner exposures to low levels in homes is not feasible because of confounding effects and significantly different dose levels.

3. Several epidemiological studies which indicate a small relative risk increase for increased residential levels appear to be subject to large errors, in particular as regards the retrospective determination of smoking habits.

4. There is substantial evidence for a threshold, or U-shaped response curve, perhaps explaining some of the beneficial effects of radon balneology. Up to about 1,000 Bq/m, lung cancer appears to be attributable to smoking only.

5. In all but very few exceptional cases, such as extremely high radon levels in the homes of heavy smokers, the cost/benefit ratio of residential radon programs does not justify the investment of private or public funds.

If considered in a larger, socio-economical and ethical context, the residential radon controversy has implications for other fields of risk/benefit assessment and regulatory control beyond radiation protection (because artificially created statistical problems obviously will not require expensive solutions). Among the serious questions to ask [20,21] are: should we really care about the potential small risks of small radiation doses which, if they exist at all, cannot yet be detected despite immense research efforts over decades? How much of a society's limited funds should be devoted to the further reduction of such hypothetical risks? How does the cost/benefit ratio of such measures compare to that for other natural and man-made hazards? How could such a degeneration of overconservative administrative concepts into serious hazards to national economies be quickly remedied (or prevented) in the future? These and many other topics clearly exceed the scope of such a brief summary.

References

1. Natural and enhanced environmental radon. Special issue of Radiat Protect Dosimet No.1, 1998.
2. Radon-Statusgespräche, Neuherberg, May 1998, and Berlin, 1999. Bonn: SSK/BMU (ISSN 09848-308X), 1998/1999.
3. Swejdemark GA. Conferences held during 1997 on indoor radon. Radiat Protect Dosimet 1998; 76:211—213.
4. Becker K. Neues zum oberirdischen Radon. Strahlenschutzpraxis (In press).
5. NRPB. Radiol Protect Bull 203 and 204;1998.
6. Mossman KL. Is indoor radon a public health hazard? The BEIR VI Report. Radiat Protect Dosimet 1998;80(4):357—360.
7. Deetjen P, Falkenbach A (eds) Radon and Health. P. Lang Verlag, (ISBN 3-631-35532-7) 1999.
8. Falkenbach A. Radon und Gesundheit. Deutsches Ärztebl 1999;96(23):1239—1240.
9. Becker K, Schüttmann W. Was ist eigentlich aus dem Radon geworden? Strahlenschutzpraxis 1998;1:54—58.
10. Schüttmann W. Bewertung des Lungenkrebsrisikos durch Wohnungsradon. Strahlenschutzpraxis 1999;5(4):35—40.
11. Conrady J et al. High residential radon health effects in Saxony (Schneeberg study). Contract F 14P-CT95-0027, European Commission, DG XII; 1999.
12. Conrady J et al. Vergleichende Analyse der räumlichen und zeitlichen Verteilung von Krebserkrankungsfällen. Dresden: Staatsminist. f. Umwelt etc., Freistaat Sachsen, 1997. See also paper, Ann Meet German Nucl Soc Munich 1998.
13. Jaggar J. Natural background radiation and cancer death in Rocky Mountain states and Gulf Coast states. Health Phys 1998;75(4):428—430.
14. Bogen KT. Mechanistic model predicts a U-shaped relation of radon exposure and lung cancer risk. Hum Exp Toxicol 1998;17:691—696.
15. Letourneau LJ. J Am Med Assoc 1987;7:578.
16. Rossi HH, Zaider M. Radiogenic lung cancer: the effect of low doses of low-LET radiation. Radiat Environ Biophys 1997;36:85—88.
17. Kellington JP et al. Effects of radiation quality on the lung cancer in CBA/Ca mice. Stratford-on-Avon: BNED London, 1997;44—51(proceedings of Internat Conf Health effects of low-level Radiat).
18. Miller RC et al. The oncogenic transformation potential of the passage of single alpha particles through mammalian cell nuclei. Proc Nat Acad Sci USA 1999;96:19—22.

19. Kreuzer M et al. Risk factors for lung cancer in young adults. Am J Epidemiol 1998;147(11): 1028—1037.
20. Becker K. How dangerous are low doses? The debate about linear vs. threshold effects. Nucl Eur Worldscan 1998;3(4):29—31. See also: Becker K, Roth R. Zur Wirkung kleiner Strahlendosen. 1998;43(10):616—620.
21. Jaworowski Z. Radiation risk and ethics. Physics Today 1999;(Sept):24—29.

High natural radiation and cancer in Karunagappally, Kerala, India

Krishnan M. Nair[1], P. Gangadharan[2], P. Jayalekshmi[2], Reghuram K. Nair[1], T. Gangadevi[1] and Jayaprakash Madhavan[1]

[1] Regional Cancer Centre, Trivandrum; and [2] Natural Background Radiation Cancer Registry, Karunagappally, India

Abstract. *Background.* The carcinogenic potential of low level chronic radiation has yet to be understood through direct observation of human populations. There are very few locations in the World where this can be done, either the radiation levels are too low or the population scarce. In a small coastal area in Kerala, a large population, almost 100,000, lives exposed to high levels of natural radiation.

Objective. To evaluate the cancer incidence in relation to exposure to natural radiation in Karunagappally taluk of Kerala.

Methods. Using house visits, total population enumeration (380,000 persons) was carried out to obtain base line data on socio-demographic lifestyle factors. The radiation exposure was measured by portable scintillometers taken from house to house (75,000 houses). A population based cancer registry recorded cancer cases in the population.

Observations and Conclusions. The radiation levels in the taluk occur with wide variations between, and within panchayat areas. Between panchayats, the median level of radiation varied from 0.918 mGy/Yr. to 5.277 mGy/Yr. When grouped and analysed as three radiation level areas, cancer incidence did not indicate any uniform elevation of incidence rates in relation to radiation levels. Greater numbers of people and more years of observation are necessary to critically evaluate the role of high natural radiation in cancer risk.

Keywords: cancer, natural radiation.

Introduction

The radiation emitting "Black Sands" of the Kerala coast have been a scientific curiosity and a health concern. A WHO expert committee (in 1957) observed that the Chavara-Neendakara coastal area in Karunagappally taluk offered great potential for radiation epidemiological studies[1]. A large population lived in the area exposed to high levels of natural radiation. The first ever epidemiological study of cancer in the area was initiated from 01-01-1990 by the Regional Cancer Centre, Trivandrum.

Address for correspondence: P. Gangadharan MSc, MS, Cancer Registry, Regional Cancer Centre, Trivandrum-695 011, Kerala, India. Tel.: +91-0471-550782, +91-0471-442541. Fax: +91-0471-550782, 91-0471-447454. E-mail: rcctvm@md2.vsnl.net.in

Objectives of the study

The objective of the study was to evaluate the relation between the chronic low-level radiation exposure and cancer as they occur in the population of the taluk.
  The study area viz.: Karunagappally taluk has the following features:

Location: Karunagappally Taluk, in Kollam District, 100 km north of Trivandrum, capital of Kerala State

Area: 192 km

Population (91 census) [2]:
               385,103 (Males:191,149) (Females:193,954)

Population density:
               2000 per sq.km

Annual growth rate:
               1.09% (1981 to 1991)

Administrative units in the Taluk:
               12 panchayats

Literacy rate: >85%

Occupation of people:
               Agriculture, Sea fishing, Fish processing factory, Coir making, Farm labourers, Cashew nut factory

Census classification:
               Rural area

Coast line: About 25 kms from south to north

Source of radiation:
               Thorium in Monazite sands of coastal area. Monazite is 1% of coastal sands of which 8−10% is Thorium

Population living in high radiation zone:
               100,000

  Migration to and from the taluk is almost negligible. People have been residing in the taluk for several centuries. The area is lush with green vegetation and typical tropical flora/fauna.

Material and Methods

The total population of the taluk was enumerated by house to house visits and information on socio-demographic and lifestyle factors were obtained on a pre-designed pro forma. The survey of the total taluk was completed over a period of 8 years during which around 380,000 people were enumerated, 66,000 inside house and 75,000 outside house radiation level measurements were taken (by a team of 14 field enumerators). The instruments and technology for radiation level measurements were guided by the Bhabha Atomic Research Centre, Mumbai. Radiation levels were measured inside and outside of every house by portable scintillometers. Inside house measurements were carried out in the living room at a height of 1 m, and outside house levels were measured in front of the entrance to the house. Thermoluminiscent dosimetric measurements were conducted in 406 houses and the annual dose recorded was compared with the estimated annual dose from spot scintillometer readings. The correlation between the two readings was $r > 0.98$. An ongoing population based cancer registry records all cancer cases occurring in the population from 01-01-1990 (according to standard methods). Cancer incidence rates were calculated by the Standard methods, and the incidence rates of cancer in Karunagappally observed from 1991 to 1992 have been published in Cancer Incidence in Five Continents Volume VII by I.A.R.C. [3].

Observations

The observations made during the period 1990 to 1998 are presented in this paper. The Karunagappally taluk is divided into 12 panchayats, which are admin-

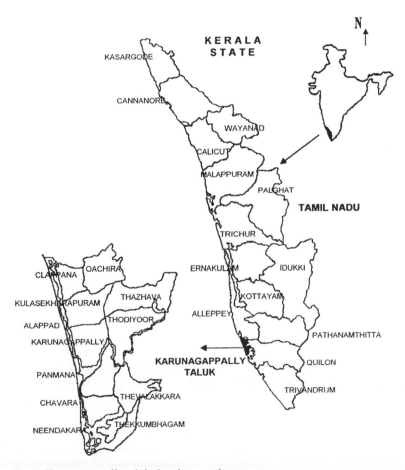

Fig. 1. Karunagappally taluk showing panchayats.

istrative units. The location of the taluk and its division into twelve panchayats are shown in Fig. 1. The radiation levels showed great heterogeneity in the different areas of every panchayat. A median radiation level (outside house) for each panchayat area was obtained from the distribution of radiation levels outside houses. Between the 12 panchayat areas these median levels varied from 0.918 mGy/yr to 5.277 mGy/yr. There are areas in the taluk where the radiation level was as high as 70 mGy/yr. Due to the wide variations between and within areas (and in order to have a reasonably homogeneous level of exposure group) the 12 panchayats were considered as 3 areas, each with 4 panchayats grouped on the basis of the median level of radiation. 2291 cancer cases were recorded as incident cancer for the 7 years, 1990—1996. The cancer incidence rates were obtained for these 3 areas from these data. The crude rate and the age-standardized rates of the three areas were obtained and are shown in Table 1 along with the range of median levels. In Tables 2 and 3, the age adjusted incidence rates of the 10 leading solid tumour sites in the 3 radiation level areas are given for males and females. In Table 4 the age adjusted incidence rates of haemopoietic malignancies (ICD 200—208) are given for both sexes.

Table 1. External γ-radiation levels (median mGy/yr) and cancer incidence rates in three grouped areas, Karunagappally taluk 1990 to 1996.

Panchayats	Incidence rates					
	Male			Female		
	CR	AAR	TAR	CR	AAR	TAR
1. Neendakara, Chavara, Panmana, Alappad. Range of Radiation level (median) mGy/yr.: [3.212—5.277]	85.2	99.4 (5.10)	179.4	69.3	79 (4.5)	160.0
2. Thekkumbhagam, Karunagappally, Clappana, Kulasheskarapuram. Range of radiation level (median) mGy/yr.: [1.835—3.059]	88.3	98.4 (5.08)	182.3	68.2	72.4 (4.18)	145.2
3. Thazhava, Thevalakkara, Thodiyoor, Oachira. Range of radiation level (median) mGy/yr.: [0.918—1.377]	91.5	102.1 (4.84)	186.8	71.5	75.9 (4.10)	150.3

Note: CR = Crude incidence rate; AAR = age adjusted rate (world population); TAR = truncated adjusted rate (35.64 years); ( ) = standard error.

Table 2. Age adjusted (world population) incidence rates of 10 leading solid tumours seen in three grouped areas in Karunagappally taluk 1990 to 1996 (male).

1. Neendakara, Chavara, Panmana, Alappad.		2. Thekkumbhagom, Karunagappally, K.S. Puram, Clappana.		3. Thazhava, Thevalakkara, Thodiyoor, Oachira.	
Lung	16.5	Lung	17.0	Lung	16.3
Stomach	6.1	Larynx	5.9	Other mouth	7.3
Oesophagus	4.3	Stomach	5.5	Stomach	6.1
Other mouth	3.9	Oesophagus	5.1	Tongue	3.0
Tongue	3.8	Other mouth	4.6	Oesophagus	5.7
Liver	3.7	Liver	4.6	Pancreas	3.6
Larynx	3.5	Uri. bladder	3.7	Prostate	3.3
Prostate	3.4	Tongue	3.5	Hypopharynx.	2.5
Brain	3.3	Oropharynx.	3.2	Uri bladder	2.5
Hypopharynx.	3.3	Prostate	2.6	Brain	2.4

Table 3. Age adjusted (world population) incidence rates of 10 leading tumours seen in three grouped areas in Karunagappally taluk 1990 to 1996 (female).

1. Neendakara, Chavara, Panmana, Alappad.		2. Thekkumbhagom, Karunagappally, K.s. Puram, Clappana.		3. Thazhava, Thevalakkara, Thodiyoor, Oachira.	
Cervix	17.4	Breast	13.9	Breast	14.3
Breast	12.5	Cervix	13.6	Cervix	13.5
Thyroid	5.0	Thyroid	3.9	Other mouth	4.2
Oesophagus	4.0	Lung	3.5	Ovary	3.4
Tongue	3.6	Ovary	3.3	Thyroid	3.2
Stomach	3.1	Oesophagus	2.7	Brain	3.0
Lung	2.3	Brain	2.4	Tongue	2.7
Brain	2.2	Other mouth	2.3	Lung	2.6
Other mouth	2.1	Stomach	2.1	Oesophagus	1.3
Ovary	1.5	Skin (non.Mel)	1.6		

Discussion

This preliminary analysis does not indicate any uniform elevation of cancer incidence rate with regard to radiation levels. As the radiation levels show wide variations between, and within panchayat areas, further studies are necessary to identify appropriate groups with uniform radiation level exposures. Dosimetric studies are continuing, however, these not only have to overcome the radiation level variations between areas but also recognise the house occupancy and mobility factor. A great majority of the population living in the high radiation coast are fishermen. The males go into the sea or spend time on the beach. More person-years of observations have to be accrued before cancer incidence data are adequately analyzed with regard to radiation levels. It is also necessary to evalu-

Table 4. Age standardise incidence rates of lymphomas and leukemias in three areas in Karunagappally taluk 1990 to 1996.

ICD-9		Male			Female		
		1.	2.	3.	1.	2.	3.
200	Lymphosarc.	1.3	1.6	3.0	0.2	0.6	0.1
201	Hodgkins d.	0.6	0.4	0.0	0.0	0.2	0.6
202	Oth. lymph.	1.2	2.4	1.4	0.5	0.3	0.7
203	Mult. myel.	0.8	1.2	0.9	0.3	1.0	0.6
204	Leuk. lympha	1.8	1.9	2.1	0.6	1.5	1.6
205	Leuk. myelo.	1.9	0.7	0.9	1.0	0.3	1.0
206	Leuk. monoc.	0.0	0.0	0.0	0.0	0.0	0.2
207	Leuk. misc.	0.0	0.0	0.0	0.0	0.0	0.0
208	Leuk. uns.	0.8	0.7	0.2	0.2	0.8	0.0

Note: 1. = Neendakara, Chavara, Panmana, Alappad; 2. = Thekkumbhagom, Karunagappally, Kulasekhara Puram (K.S. Puram), Clappana; 3. = Thazhava, Thevalakkara, Thodiyoor, Oachira.

ate the risk levels in the presence of known high risk factors for cancer such as tobacco habits etc. which would be competing risk factors in this context. It is also of paramount interest to pursue biological studies into the different radiation dose levels and dose-rate levels. The present study has obtained the essential base line data in this regard.

Table 1 indicates that in terms of area, no marked differences in overall cancer incidence has been noted. Tables 2 and 3 also show little evidence that the incidence is related to radiation levels. Among men, lung cancer has a higher rate in all of the areas than other types. Among females, cervix cancer alone has higher rate in area 1 compared to the other areas. In area 1, the socio-cultural risk factors (especially that of deprivation) may be in operation.

Conclusions

As the population has been living in the area for decades, the lack of any large increase in incidence rates indicates that:
a) no association with the radiation levels present in the area;
b) very low elevated or reduced risk which was not detectable by simple analysis and due to the small size of the population study; or
c) variations in the prevalence of other high risk factors in different areas which confounds or competes with the effect of radiation exposure. Further studies are thus essential.

Acknowledgements

We wish to acknowledge the financial support of B.R.N.S. (No.4/10/89) for this study as well as the technical support given by the E.A.D., Health Physics Division B.A.R.C., Medical Doctors in Karunagappally, Doctors in Regional Cancer Centre, the Panchayats and the general public of Karunagappally, who have wholeheartedly cooperated with us in this project. It is our pleasure to express our thanks to Dr U.C. Mishra, Director of Health, Safety and Environment, B.A.R.C. for supporting this study.

References

1. Gopal–Ayengar AR. Possible areas with sufficiently different background radiation levels to permit detection of differences of mutation rates of marker genes. In: Effect of Radiation on Human Heredity. Geneva: WHO, 1957;115–124.
2. Final population totals, Paper 3 of 1991, Director of Census Operations. Kerala, 1991.
3. Parkin DM, Whelam SL, Ferlay J, Raymond L, Young J (eds) Cancer Incidence in Five Continents Vol. VII. I.A.R.C. Scientific Publication No.143, 1997.

Genetic epidemiological studies in the high level natural radiation (HLNR) areas of Kerala in the south west coast of India

G. Jaikrishan[1], V.D. Cheriyan[1], C.J. Kurien[1], V.J. Andrews[1], Birajalaxmi Das[1],
E.N. Ramachandran[1], C.V. Karuppasamy[1], D.C. Soren[1], M.V. Thampi[1],
P.K.M. Koya[1], V.K. Rajan[2] and P.S. Chauhan[1]

[1]Monazite Survey Project, Cell Biology Division, Bhabha Atomic Research Centre, Trombay; and [2]Directorate of Health Services, Government of Kerala, Thiruvananthapuram, India

Abstract. The densely populated monazite-bearing high level natural radiation (HLNR) areas of the Kerala coast (with annual radiation dose rates ranging from 1.0 to over 40.0 Gy), provide unique opportunities for investigating the health effects of low-level chronic radiation directly in human populations. As a part of the programme on assessment of biological and health effects of this radiation exposure in humans, the monitoring of newborns is being undertaken to determine the incidence of malformations and constitutional chromosome abnormalities. Currently available data on the screening of 47,643 newborns for malformations (and cytogenetic analysis of 18,784 newborns) are reported in this communication.

The monitoring for malformations is being undertaken in four hospitals located in the study area, where each newborn is screened for malformations at birth. For chromosomal studies, cord blood samples are brought to the field laboratory and processed for chromosomal analysis.

Among the total 47,643 newborns, there were 251 (0.53%) stillborns, 340 twin births, three triplets, and one set of quadruplets. The overall incidence of malformation was 1.65% and showed a maternal age dependent increase. The stillborns exhibited a very high malformation rate of 23.11% compared to some 1.53% among liveborns. The twin births also had a higher malformation rate of 2.21% compared to that of the singletons (1.64%). Thirty-eight cases of Down syndrome (DS) were identified with an incidence of 1 in 1,249 births. Babies born of consanguneous marriages (3.0%) too had a relatively higher rate of malformations (2.23%) as well as still births (1.04%). About 92% of deliveries took place before the mother's maternal age of 29 years. The the number of newborns from HLNR and normal level radiation (NLNR) areas was 34,337 and 13,306, respectively. The overall incidence of still births, malformations, and DS in the newborns from HLNR areas was 0.56, 1.69, and 0.087%, respectively; which wwas comparable with values of 0.44, 1.53, and 0.060%, respectively, from NLNR areas. The cytogenetic analysis of 18,784 newborns (5,086 from NLNR and 13,698 from HLNR) for constitutional chromosomal anomalies has so far been completed. The observed incidence of constitutional anomalies 5.00 ± 0.52 per 1,000 newborns is similar to that reported elsewhere. The total autosomal and sex chromosome aneuploids, as well as structrural anomalies, were comparable between HLNR and NLNR areas and did not show any association with the background radiation levels.

The data available so far with respect to congenital malformations and constitutional chromosomal anomalies does not reveal any effect that can be associated with radiation exposure. The studies are in progress to build an adequate database required for individual malformations and chromosomal variants to draw statistically valid conclusions in this controversial area of the health effects of low-level radiation in human populations.

Address for correspondence: Dr M. Seshadri, Project Manager, Monazite Survey Project, Bhabha Atomic Research Center, Trombay Mumbai – 400 085, India. Tel.: +91-22-5505139. Fax: +91-22-5505151. E-mail: msesh@apsara.barc.ernet.in

Introduction

The biological and health effects of low-level radiation in humans continues to be a subject of debate. Available estimates of the genetic effects in humans at low doses of radiation exposure are based on linear extrapolation (downward) to a zero dose level from the effects observed at high doses (of acute radiation) in laboratory animals (and very limited data in humans). Uncertainties inherent with the assumptions of extrapolation, and recent evidence of radio-adaptive responses in mammalian cells including human lymphocytes, emphasises the need for direct human studies at low-dose and low dose-rate exposures [1]. The populations living in the high level natural radiation (HLNR) areas of the southwest coast of Kerala, exposed to chronic low-level radiation for several generations provide unique opportunities for elucidating the effects of low level exposure directly in humans. The radioactivity in this monazite belt is primarily due to Thorium (and decay products) constituting 8 to 10% of the black sands. The radioactivity in different areas is high, varying from 1.0 mGy to over 40.0 mGy/year [2—4]. In view of the above, a field laboratory was established in the area by the research centre and a comprehensive programme launched to investigate the biological and health effects of low level radiation in humans living in the area. Ionizing radiations are well known to induce chromosomal and/or gene mutations in somatic as well as germ cells in a wide variety of organisms. Screening of newborns for phenotypic variants and chromosomal/gene mutations at birth is perhaps the most practical approach to determine the extent of genetic damage in the human population. Studies on the monitoring of the newborns, for major congenital malformations and constitutional chromosomal anomalies, which form a part of the health assessment programme being undertaken by the field laboratory are summerized in this communication.

Materials and Methods

The studies are being carried out in collaboration with the Department of Health, Government of Kerala, responsible for the public health in the state. In the four state Government hospitals catering to the study population, all the newborns are monitored for major congenital malformations identifiable at birth [5]. Data pertaining to socio-demographic profile, pregnancy history, life style, occupation, consanguinity, place of stay of the parents etc. are elucidated from the family and recorded according to the pro forma designed under WHO guidelines. The completeness and consistency of information is ascertained at different levels and further verified prior to inclusion in the computer database. The average radiation levels for the family are incorporated in case of each newborn. The data entry is verified and validated for internal consistency.

For cytogenetic studies, cord blood samples (collected in sterile heparinised vials from consecutive births from the two hospital units of the study areas) are transported to the field laboratory, the low level radiation research laboratory

(LLRRL), in refrigerated conditions. The whole blood cultures are set up using standard procedures [6] as reported by Cheriyan et al. in their recent report [7]. In each culture tube, 0.4 ml of cord blood was grown in 4 ml of nutrient mixture F-10 HAM supplemented with 5 percent 200 mM L-Glutamine, to which was added 10 percent foetal calf serum and 2 percent phytohemagglutinin and terminated at 48 h by the addition of 0.04 µg/ml Colcemid. The coded slides stained in Giemsa (G-banded wherever necessary) were analysed by a group of five to six cytogeneticists and karyotyping 20 cells are visually karyotyped per sample. Each numerical and structural chromosomal abnormality is confirmed by at least three or more cytogeneticists before being recorded. Radiation measurements are taken from all the four sides of the households using a radiation meter. The present radiation measurements are in conformity with the detailed dosimetry studies carried out earlier [2–4]. The average radiation dose in control areas of the Quilon district is 1.2 mGy per year with a range of < 1.0–1.5 mGy per year. Hence, areas with a radiation exposure above 1.5 mGy per year are considered as HLNR areas and those with below 1.5 mGy/year, as normal level natural radiation (NLNR) areas. The classification of HLNR and NLNR is based on the radiation level prevailing at the residence of the mother and provides the opportunity to have in-built controls. Though the mobility of the population is an important factor, a high correlation between the average dose rates and the observed dose-rates in air from terrestrial γ-radiation both in the outdoors and indoors of the study area lends support to the classification.

Statistical analysis

The proportion of newborns with congenital anomalies across various subgroups was compared by using χ^2 test. The comparison of the prevalence in HLNR and NLNR areas was made by using the "Relative Risk" (relative frequency) approach. The significance of the observed relative frequency (RF) was judged from the confidence interval (CI). RF is statistically significant if the CI does not include one, which is the value of RF under the null hypothesis of there existing no difference between HLNR and NLNR areas [8]. To eliminate the possible effects of confounding factors, a stratified analysis was also carried out. In the case of chromosome variants a Poisson distribution was assumed.

Results

During these studies (from a total of 47,643 newborns examined so far) 784 newborns have been identified as having malformations, exhibiting an incidence of 1.65% at birth (Table 1). The prevalence of malformations among 251 (0.53%) still borns was almost 15-fold higher at 23.11%. The twins also exhibited relatively higher malformation rates. Consanguinity resulted in higher risk of malformations as well as still births (Table 2). The incidence of malformations was found to be associated with maternal age. The male child was at a significantly

Table 1. Genetic epidemiological studies in the HLNR areas of Kerala: congenital malformations, still births and twinning.

Newborns	Normal	Malformed	Total	Malformed (%)
Total newborns	46859	784	47643	1.65
Live births	46666	726	47392	1.53
Still births	193	58	251 (0.53)	23.11
Singletons	46181	769	46950	1.64
Live births	46010	715	46725	1.53
Still births	171	54	225 (0.48)	24.00
Twins	665	15	680	2.21
Live births	645	11	656	1.68
Still births	20	4	24 (3.53)	16.67
Multiples				
(3 Triplets, 1 Quadruplet)	13	–	13	–
Live births	11	–	11	–
Still births	2	–	2 (15.38)	–

Note: Figures in parenthesis denote the percentage of the respective event. Still births include intra-uterine deaths, still births, and those born alive but died immediately without any physical stress. Malformations were more common among still births ($p < 0.001$). Radiation dose rate in the area ranges from 7 to 550 $\mu R/h$ or to about 0.6 to 48.2 mGy/year, with an overall mean of 2.39 mGy/year.

higher risk of malformation compared to the female counterparts (1.99 vs. 1.26%, $p < 0.05$), mainly due to the anomalies of the male urogenital system, such as cryptorchidism and hypospadiasis. As many as 92% of the babies born were to mothers below (and including) the age of 29, and only 1.2% above the maternal age of 34 years (Table 2). The major religious groups in the study population are Hindus (68.1%), followed by Muslims (19.7%) and Christians (12.1%). The incidence of malformations among different ethnic groups of Hindus showed variation ranging from 1.42% among Nairs to 2.36% among Arayas, with an overall frequency of 1.63%. It is noteworthy that the Araya ethnic group (1.5% of the total population) also exhibited the highest rate of consanguineous marriages (6.6%). Traditionally fishermen, the Araya Muslims live in the coastal areas where radiation levels are also relatively quite high (about 68% of Arayas are exposed to a dose rate of more than 6 mGy per year). The least incidence of malformations was among the Christians, incidentally the group with lowest proportion of consanguineous marriages (0.96%). The incidence of malformations showed no association with radiation levels (Table 3) and was comparable between HLNR and NLNR areas (1.69 vs. 1.53%; RF of 1.08, 95% CI: 0.90 to 1.31). Thirty-eight cases of Down syndrome (DS) were identified, with an incidence of one in 1254 births. The incidence increased with maternal age, the frequency being one cas of DS in 3307, 1529, 1996, and 300 births, respectively, in the maternal age groups of 15—19, 20—24, 25—29, and $\geqslant$ 30 years (Trend χ^2

Table 2. Genetic epidemiological studies in the HLNR areas of Kerala: congenital malformations, still births, consanguinity and maternal age.

Characteristics	Total births		Malformations		Still births	
	No.	(%)	No.	(%)	No.	(%)
Total	47643	100	784	1.65	251	0.53
Consanguinity						
Absent	46205	97.0	752	1.63	236	0.51
Preset	1438	3.0	32	2.23	15	1.04
Gender						
Male	24562	51.6	490	1.99	138	0.56
Female	23078	48.4	291	1.26	112	0.49
Intersex	3		3		1	
Maternal age						
15–19	3307	6.9	49	1.48	24	0.73
20–24	24464	51.3	406	1.66	110	0.45
25–29	15970	33.5	244	1.52	84	0.53
30–34	3351	7.0	73	2.18	26	0.78
⩾ 35	551	1.2	12	2.18	7	1.27
Religion						
Hindu	32461	68.1	430	1.63	170	0.52
Christian	5782	12.1	82	1.42	28	0.48
Muslim	9400	19.7	172	1.83	53	0.56
Radiation area						
High-level (> 1.50 mGy/y)	34337	72.1	580	1.69	193	0.56
Low-level (⩽ 1.50 mGy/y)	13306	27.9	204	1.53	58	0.44

Note: Radiation dose rate in the area ranges from 7 to 550 μR/h or 0.6 to 48.2 mGy/year, with an average of 2.39 mGy/year. The average doses for high and low-level radiation areas were 2.85 and 1.21 mGy/year, respectively. The difference in the incidence of malformation among males and females is statistically significant ($p < 0.001$) and is largely due to malformations associated with male uro-genital system. The frequencies of still births in different age groups are not similar ($p < 0.01$). Still births are more common among consanguineous marriages ($p < 0.05$).

34.9, $p < 0.001$).

The cytogenetic studies have been going on since 1986 in the study area, studies which involved both screening for chromosomal aberrations as well as visual karyotyping for constitutional anomalies. As reported earlier [7] a total of 963,940 metaphases from 10,230 newborns were analysed for various types of chromosomal aberration, with 8,493 newborns (804,212 cells) from HLNR areas (average dose rate 4.5 mGy/y) and 1,737 newborns (159,728 cells) from NLNR (average dose rate 1.15 mGy/y). Unstable chromosomal aberrations such as dicentrics (with and without fragments), rings, fragments, and breaks as well as stable configurations including translocations and inversions were scored from

Table 3. Genetic epidemiological studies in the HLNR areas of Kerala: dose-rate and malformations.

Radiation dose		Total		Newborns with malformation		Relative frequency	
(mGy/year)	Mean	No.	(%)	No.	(%)		
$\leqslant$ 1.50	1.21[a]	13306	29.7	204	1.53	1.00	
1.51−3.00	1.80	29717	62.4	506	1.70	1.11	(0.95−1.31)
3.01−6.00	4.09	2821	5.9	40	1.42	0.92	(0.66−1.29)
6.01−18.00	13.64	1288	2.7	24	1.86	1.22	(0.80−1.85)
$\geqslant$ 18.01	29.67	511	1.1	10	1.96	1.27	(0.68−2.39)
Total	2.39	47643	100.0	784	1.65		

Note: [a]Mean radiation levels in the respective group; the lowest and highest radiation levels recorded in the area were 0.70 and 48.18 mGy/year; () = denote lower and upper limits of 95% confidence intervals (CI).

coded slides. None of the aberrations showed any radiation to have any relationship with the radiation levels prevalent in the area. The karyotyping analysis based on 20 metaphases continues to establish the frequency of constitutional anomalies in the population. The 18,784 newborns screened cytogenetically for constitutional anomalies include 12,496 newborns from HLNR and 3,673 from NLNR areas. Ninety four newborns with constitutional chromosome anomalies were identified with a frequency of 5.11 ± 0.61 per 1,000 newborns. These included 50 numerical and 44 structural chromosomal variants (Table 4). The numerical variants included 16 cases of Down syndrome, two Patau's, three Edward's syndromes, one double aneuploid, four triple X, eight Klinefelter's, three Turner's syndromes, nine XYY, and four with additional centric fragments, with an overall frequency of 2.66 ± 0.38 per 1,000 newborns. Structural anomalies (2.34 ± 0.35 per 1,000) included six deletions, eight inversions, 11 Robertsonian translocations, and 19 with other translocations. There were no significant differences between HNLR and NLNR areas in the incidence of total constitutional anomalies.

Discussion

With the realization of the unique opportunity of investigating biological and health effects of low level radiation in this region several studies have been undertaken in the past. These include dosimetric measurements of radiation levels in the area [2−4] and cytogenetic studies on native plants belonging to different genera and species [9−10]. The genetic studies in wild rats based on skeletal and dental variants [11,12] showed no radiation associated effects. In humans, a demographic study in a population of 70,000 individuals also showed no significant differences in reproductive parameters, infant mortality etc. between the high and normal level radiation areas [13]. However, a higher prevalence of

Table 4. Genetic epidemiological studies in the HLNR areas of Kerala: constitutional chromosomal abnormalities among newborns.

Abnormality	Total (n = 18784)		High level natural radiation area (n = 13698)		Normal level natural radiation area (n = 5086)	
	No.	Frequency (f)	No.	f	No.	f
Numerical autosomal trisomies	21	1.12 ± 0.24	15	1.10 ± 0.28	6	1.18 ± 0.48
48,XXY + 21	1	0.05 ± 0.05	1	0.07 ± 0.07	—	—
+Centric fragments	4 (2 mosaics)	0.21 ± 0.11	3 (1 mosaic)	0.22 ± 0.13	1 (1 mosaic)	0.20 ± 0.20
Sex chromosomal	24 (9 mosaics)	1.28 ± 0.26	20 (6 mosaics)	1.46 ± 0.33	4 (3 mosaics)	0.79 ± 0.39
Total numerical	50	2.66 ± 0.38	39	2.85 ± 0.46	11	2.16 ± 0.65
Structural deletion	6	0.32 ± 0.13	3	0.22 ± 0.13	3	0.59 ± 0.34
Inversion	8	0.43 ± 0.15	7	0.51 ± 0.19	1	0.20 ± 0.20
Robertsonian translocation	11	0.59 ± 0.18	7	0.51 ± 0.19	4	0.79 ± 0.39
Other translocations	19	1.01 ± 0.23	14	1.02 ± 0.27	5	0.98 ± 0.44
Total structral	44	2.34 ± 0.35	31	2.26 ± 0.41	13	2.56 ± 0.71
Overall	94	5.00 ± 0.52	70	5.11 ± 0.61	24	4.72 ± 0.96

Note: High level natural radiation area = dose > 1.50 mGy/year; normal level natural radiation area = dose ≤ 1.50 mGy/year, average 4.36 mGy/year; normal level natural radiation area = dose ≤ 1.50 mGy/year, average 1.14 mGy/year; n = sample size; No. = number of samples with the abnormality; frequency = per / 1,000; SE = standard error, assuming Poisson distribution.

Down syndrome among population from HLNR area was claimed by Kochupillai et al. [14], with no DS case having been recorded in the control population. The Department of Atomic Energy (BARC) established a field laboratory in the area to study in depth the biological and health effects of the high level radiation on human population, with major emphasis on the genetic effects. This programme includes the monitoring of the newborns for congenital malformations and chromosomal anomalies as well as a demographic health survey and cytogenetic studies among the adult population.

   Unlike the other parts of India, the population in the study area is generally literate, health conscious, and practices small family norms. The mean maternal age of 24.2 years at delivery was low with only 8% of the deliveries occurring after the age of 30 years. Primi together with second-gravida constituted 90% of the births. The rate of still births was also comparatively lower at 0.58% than the rest of the country and so was the rate of low birthweight babies (< 2,500 g), at 7.5%. The sex ratio (M:F) among twin births was 1000:1105 as compared to 1000:937 among singleton deliveries, probably supporting the hypothesis of the role of X inactivation in the process of twinning of female zygotes [15] and consequent preponderance of female monozygotic twins. As expected, the incidence of DS showed a maternal-age dependent increase, with an overall frequency of 1 DS per 1,254 births. The relatively lower incidence is compatible with the younger maternal age as reported recently [16,17]. The present number of 38 DS cases is too small to draw conclusive dose-response relationships from (with such wide variation in radiation dose rates). However, the limited data available so far shows no significant differences between newborns from HLNR and NLNR areas, nor was there any association with different radiation levels. These observations stand in contrast to the report of Kochupillai et al. [14] which was based on a population survey. These investigations were beset by the problem of the absence of any DS child within normal radiation (control) areas. There was also no maternal age dependency. In a recently concluded multicentric Down syndrome study, the overall frequency of DS in the Indian population was found to be 1 in 1,139 births with clear maternal-age dependency (project report submitted by Verma, Anand, Modi and Bharucha to BRNS, DAE, 1999). The incidence of DS in the comparative maternal age group (of the multicentric study) was comparable to that of our present study. The multicentric study, however, had a higher number of deliveries above the maternal age of 35 years compared with that of the Kerala population. Thus, the incidence of DS in Indian population from control (NLNR) areas further highlights the weakness of the claims made by Kochupillai et al. as discussed by ourselves [5] and by other investigators [18].

   In the cytogenetic studies almost all types of constitutional chromosomal abnormality reported in the literature were observed among the newborns of this study. The classical syndromes involving autosomes were typical trisomies with no mosaics noted. However, mosaics were observed in sex chromosomal anomalies in addition to trisomies (except in the cases of Turner syndrome). All the 16 Down syndrome (DS) cases were primary trisomy 21. The overall incidence of DS (one in 1,174 births) represents the study population. There were no significant differences among newborns from high and normal levels of radiation with respect to DS and other autosomal or sex aneuploids. Thus the cytogenetic analysis of newborns at birth also contrasts the claim of higher DS cases in HLNR areas [14]. The overall incidence of constitutional chromosomal anomalies (5.00 ± 0.52 per 1,000 newborns) is comparable with published literature [1]. It must be emphasized that the incidence of congenital malformations and/or chromosomal constitutional anomalies at the various radiation dose rates is based on limited data, especially at higher radiation levels where only a large sample size with adequate numbers would provide reliable conclusions. However, the observations corroborate with the genetic studies on the children of parents exposed during the atomic bombing of Hiroshima and Nagasaki, which also showed no statistically significant differences to the unexposed groups [19]. In a recent study on cancer epidemiology in the studied population of Kerala, the age standardized cancer rates involving large population groups have also failed to show any association with radiation background levels [20], and the overall cancer prevalence was comparable with the rest of the Kerala state. The Chinese studies in HLNR areas (based on 32 disorders) have also shown no increase in congenital malformations associated with radiation levels [21]. In conclusion, based on the data available so far, no significant differences in the incidence of malformations and/or constitutional chromosomal anomalies in the newborns from HLNR and NLNR areas were observed. The programme continues so as to obtain an adequate sample size for statistically valid conclusions and in order to address some of the issues surrounding the controversial area of health effects of low level radiation exposure in humans.

Acknowledgements

The authors are grateful for the enoromous help and unfailing support of the Department of Health of Kerala state, particularly the collaborating medical and paramedical staff of the four hospitals catering to the study area. Without their dedication and hard work, these investigations would not have been possible. We are thankful to K.P. Bhaskaran, R. Prabhakaran and P.S. Mohan for excellent technical assistance rendered during the cytogenetic studies. Thanks are also due to P.N. Panicker and the other technical staff of our laboratory who have contributed to these studies in many ways. The authors are also indebtcd to Doctor's M. Seshadri and K.B. Sainis for their suggestions and encouragement.

References

1. UNSCEAR (United Nations Scientific Committee on the Effects of Atomic Radiation). Report to the General Assembly. New York: United Nations, 1993.

194

2. Bharatwal DS, Vaze GH. Radiation dose measurements in the monazite areas of Kerala state in India. Peaceful uses of Atomic Energy, Geneva: United Nations, 1958;23:156(proceedings of the 2nd UN international conference).
3. Sunta CM. A review of the studies of high background areas of the southwest coast of India. In: Sohrabi M, Ahmed JU, Durani SA (eds). Tehran, Iran: Atomic Energy Organization of Iran, 1993;71(proceedings of the International conference on high levels of natural radiation).
4. Mistry KB, Bhathran KG, Gopal Ayengar AR. Radioactivity in the diet of population of Kerala coast including monazite bearing high radiation areas. Health Phys 1970;19:535—542.
5. Jaikrishan G, Andrews VJ, Thampi MV, Koya PKM, Rajan VK, Chauhan PS. Genetic monitoring of human population from high-level natural radiation areas of Kerala on the southwest coast of India. I. Prevalence of congenital malformations in newborns. Radiat Res 1999;152(Suppl):S149—S153.
6. Moorhead PS, Nowell PC, Mellman WJ, Battips DM, Hungerford DA. Chromosome preparations of leukocytes cultured from human peripheral blood. Exp Cell Res 1960;20:613—616.
7. Cheriyan VD, Kurien CJ, Das B, Ramachandran EN, Karuppasamy CV, Thampi MV, George KP, Kesavan PC, Koya PKM, Chauhan PS. Genetic monitoring of human population from high-level natural radiation areas of Kerala on the Southwest Coast of India. II. Incidence of numerical and structural chromosomal aberrations in the lymphocytes of newborns. Radiat Res 1999;152(Suppl):S154—S158.
8. Kahn HA, Sempos CT. Statistical Methods in Epidemiology. Oxford University Press, 1989.
9. Gopala Ayengar AR, Nayar GG, George KP, Mistry KB. Biological effects of high background radioactivity - studies on plants growing on the monazite bearing areas of Kerala coast and adjourning regions. Indian J Exp Biol 1970;8.
10. Nayar GG, George KP, Gopal Ayengar AR. On the biological effects of high background radioactivity: studies on tradascantia grown in radioactive monazite sand. Radiat Bot 1970;10: 287—292.
11. Gruneberg H. Genetical research in an area of high natural radioactivity in South India. Nature 1964;204:222—224.
12. Gruneberg H, Bains GH, Berry RJ, Riles L, Smith CAB, Weiss RA. A search for genetic effects of high natural radioactivity in South India. In: Report SRS 307. London: Medical Research Council, Her Majesty's Stationary Office, 1966.
13. Gopal-Ayengar AR, Sundaram K, Mistry KB, Suntha CM, Nambi KSV, Kaithuria SP, Basu AS, David M. Evaluation of the long term effects of high background radiation on selected population groups of Kerala coasts. In: Peaceful uses of Atomic Energy. Geneva: United Nations, 1971;31—61(proceeding IV of the 2nd UN international conference).
14. Kochupillai N, Verma IC, Grewal MS, Ramalingaswamy V. Down syndrome and related abnormalities in an area of high background radiation in coastal Kerala. Nature 1976;262: 60—61.
15. Phelan MC. Twins. In: Stevenson RE, Hall JG, Goodman RM (eds) Human Malformations and Related Anomalies Vol II. New York: Oxford University Press, 1993.
16. Hecht CA, Hook EB. Rates of Down syndrome at live birth by one-year maternal age intervals in studies with apparent close to complete ascertainment in populations of European origin: a proposed revised rate schedule for use in genetic and prenatal screening. Am J Med Gen 1996; 62:376—385.
17. Carothers AD, Boyd E, Lowther G, Ellis PM, Couzin DA, Faed MJW, Robb A. Trends in prenatal diagnosis of Down syndrome and other autosomal trisomies in Scotland 1990 to 1994, with associated cytogenetic and epidemiological findings. Genet Epidemiol 1999;16:179—190.
18. Rose KSB. Review of health studies in Kerala. Nucl Energy 1982;21:399—408.
19. Neel JV, Schull WJ, Awa AA, Satoh C, Kato H, Otake M, Yoshimoto Y. The children of parents exposed to atomic bombs: estimates of the genetic doubling dose of radiation for humans. Am J Hum Genet 1990;46:1053—1072.

20. Krishnan-Nair M, Nambi KSV, Sreedevi-Amma N, Gangadharan P, Jayalekshmy P, Jayadevan S, Varghese C, Raghuram K Nair. Population study in the high natural background radiation area in Kerala, India. Radiat Res 1999;152(Suppl):S145—S148.
21. Wei L, Zha Y, Tao Z, He W, Chen D, Yaun Y. Epidemilogical investigations of radiological effects in high background radiation areas of Yangjiang, China. Radiat Res 1990;31:119—136.

Index of authors

Keyword index